Whoa, Baby!

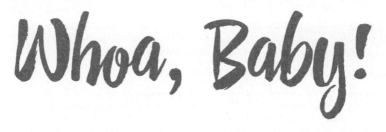

Whoa, Baby!

A GUIDE FOR NEW MOMS WHO FEEL OVERWHELMED AND FREAKED OUT

(and Wonder What the #*$& Just Happened)

Kelly Rowland

and Tristan Emily Bickman, MD
with Laura Moser

Da Capo

LIFE
LONG

Copyright © 2017 by KTR, Inc. and Dr. Tristan Emily Bickman

Library of Congress Cataloging-in-Publication Data
Names: Rowland, Kelly, 1981– author. | Bickman, Tristan Emily, author. | Moser, Laura, author.
Title: Whoa, baby! : a guide for new moms who feel overwhelmed and freaked out (and wonder what the #*$& just happened) / by Kelly Rowland and Dr. Tristan Emily Bickman with Laura Moser.
Description: Boston, MA : Da Capo Lifelong Books, [2017]
Identifiers: LCCN 2016043406 (print) | LCCN 2016044162 (ebook) |
ISBN 9780738219424 (hardback) | ISBN 9780738219431 (ebook)
Subjects: LCSH: Pregnancy—Popular works. | Childbirth—Popular works. | Women—Health and hygiene—Popular works. | Parenting—Popular works. | BISAC: HEALTH & FITNESS / Pregnancy & Childbirth. | HEALTH & FITNESS / Women's Health. | FAMILY & RELATIONSHIPS / Parenting / Motherhood.
Classification: LCC RG551 .R69 2017 (print) | LCC RG551 (ebook) | DDC 618.2—dc23
LC record available at https://lccn.loc.gov/2016043406

First Da Capo Press edition 2017

Published by Da Capo Press, an imprint of Perseus Books, LLC,
a subsidiary of Hachette Book Group, Inc.
www.dacapopress.com

Note: The information in this book is true and complete to the best of our knowledge. This book is intended only as an informative guide for those wishing to know more about health issues. In no way is this book intended to replace, countermand, or conflict with the advice given to you by your own physician. The ultimate decision concerning care should be made between you and your doctor. We strongly recommend you follow his or her advice. Information in this book is general and is offered with no guarantees on the part of the authors or Da Capo Press. The authors and publisher disclaim all liability in connection with the use of this book.

Da Capo Press books are available at special discounts for bulk purchases in the U.S. by corporations, institutions, and other organizations. For more information, please contact the Special Markets Department at the Perseus Books Group, 2300 Chestnut Street, Suite 200, Philadelphia, PA, 19103, or call (800) 810-4145, ext. 5000, or e-mail special.markets@perseusbooks.com.

Editorial production by Christine Marra, Marrathon Production Services. www.marrathoneditorial.com

DESIGN BY JANE RAESE
Set in 12-point Bulmer

10 9 8 7 6 5 4 3 2 1

TO TIM & TITAN,
My inspiration every day!
I love you! ♥
—*Kelly Rowland*

TO KELLY,
who is the best collaborator ever.

TO MY PATIENTS,
who have provided me with my passion and a lifetime of memories.

TO MY FAMILY,
especially my husband David and five amazing children,
Jacob, Matthew, Amanda, Abby, and Juliet, and
my perfect parents,
who understand and support me in every way.
I am blessed. This book is long overdue.
—*Dr. Tristan Emily Bickman*

CONTENTS

What Do I Do Now?

I am not lying when I say that I loved every second of my pregnancy. I know, I know. I was one of *those* women. I realized then and now how incredibly lucky I was in that I never felt too sick or had any major health scares. And I was so excited to become a mom. I was doing it exactly as I'd always dreamed. I was married and madly in love with my husband, Tim. I was at a great age, and a great stage in my career—established enough to be financially comfortable, with the luxury of being able to take a few months off to focus on the baby.

And pregnancy, for me, just confirmed how wonderful being a mom was guaranteed to be. I loved that even when I was relaxing, I was accomplishing something major. I was growing a baby inside my body—what could be more important than that? And I just couldn't get enough of the attention my friends and family showered on me. Everyone was always rubbing my belly and offering me the best seat on the couch and generally treating me like the queen of the world. That's exactly what I felt like: a queen!

I allowed myself more indulgences than in my regular, non-pregnant life, and I loved eating my number-one pregnancy food, chocolate ice cream with peanut butter mixed in it, several times a week. After what felt like a lifetime of monitoring my diet, I could finally eat whatever I wanted and not worry about it! (Note to self for future pregnancies: This is not actually true. But, hey, it was awesome while it lasted.)

I was so into my new queen status that I wasn't prepared for the seismic shift that took place when my son exited my body and entered the world. Right after Titan was born, we did the skin-to-skin and he squirmed around on my chest and I was in absolute heaven, surrounded by everyone I loved best on earth. But then, a few minutes later, the nurses whisked him away from me to be weighed and cleaned up. And just as suddenly, the crew who'd been cheering me on—my husband, my godsisters—literally just forgot all about me. They went, as my beloved obstetrician, Tristan Bickman, said, straight from "the 'gina to the warmer." It was true. They were just totally outta there.

My husband had been all "You rocked that birth, baby—I'm so proud of you!" But then, once Titan came out, he seemed to forget all about my accomplishment. Just like that, he was bent over Titan's tiny body whispering, "You're Daddy's champ! You're Daddy's champ!" over and over. And once everyone had followed Daddy's little champ across the room, I was left lying back in the hospital bed, all alone except for Dr. Bickman, thinking, "Hello? What about me? Aren't I a champ, too?"

Of the million different emotions—ecstatic and excited and scared to death, to name a few—swirling inside me at that life-changing moment, one thing I didn't expect to feel was abandoned. But it was as if, in the second I gave birth, my loved ones forgot all about me!

In the blink of an eye everything was all about Titan. And of course that's what it is to be a parent—that's exactly how it's supposed to be. I, too, was feeling the most incredible love I had ever experienced for that tiny little man who had just emerged from my body. But I was also feeling an incredible pain in my vajayjay and wondering if I'd ever walk again.

I'd spent nine months so focused on the baby growing inside me that I was caught completely off guard when I discovered that, over the course of my pregnancy, I had changed, too. Like many first-time moms, I'd assumed that once I popped out the baby, I'd be taking care of him and that would be that. I didn't realize how hard it would be for me to have a bowel movement or breastfeed or even sleep. That first day, for all my excitement, I was also feeling exhausted and overwhelmed and a little bewildered.

It was a good thing that Dr. Bickman, who's been my ob/gyn for the last fourteen years, was right there next to me (unlike my family members—ha!) to answer every single crazy question that popped into my head not just in those first few minutes, but in the days that followed. In those intense weeks of brand-new motherhood, I was calling up poor Dr. Bickman at every hour of the day and night, every time with a new question. While I had been completely chill throughout my pregnancy, just letting nature run its course, I suddenly had endless questions—crazy questions, nasty questions, embarrassing questions, you name it. Why do I feel even heavier after giving birth? Will I ever be able to go to the bathroom without wincing again? Why am I bleeding so damn much? What's up with falling asleep the second I start nursing? Why don't I get as wet when I see my husband when I'm still so attracted to him?

None of these questions, no matter how raunchy, fazed Dr. Bickman for one second. She provided me with the reassurance I so desperately needed, telling me over and over that, in the months after a woman gives birth, nothing is exactly strange, but nothing is necessarily normal, either. It's all just part of the "miracle" of birth. Throughout my pregnancy but even more so afterward, Dr. B. made me feel like what was happening to my body was completely natural, no matter how nasty or scary: the Frisbee boobs, the stretched-out vaj, the clumps of hair falling out every morning.

And when I spoke with her, she told me that a huge number of patients are exactly like me. They think that now that they've done the whole pregnancy thing, they can turn their attention to taking care of their newborn baby and that's that. They never consider how their own bodies might react to what they've just gone through until something goes wrong— and then, like me, they feel overwhelmed and freaked out and don't know where to turn. Every day in the weeks and months after I became a mom, it seemed like I had a new question. Why am I sweating through my sheets? What's up with all this hair falling out? Will I ever be able to have sex again? Will I ever even want to?

Even if you think you're the first woman in the history of the world to confront a specific post-pregnancy concern, trust me, you're not. Just because we don't talk about these subjects at cocktail parties or mommy-and-me classes doesn't make them less real, or less common. That's why every new mom out there needs a Dr. Bickman in their life: a kind, hilarious, and wise woman who has seen everything and then some. Every time I called her in the weeks after Titan arrived on the scene, I was sure she'd be shocked or horrified or just grossed out by whatever I had to ask her. But more often than not, she'd heard it before, and not just once, but often that same day!

Dr. Bickman was the perfect person to answer all my questions because she has been there and done that. She has five kids of her own ranging in age from four to eighteen, and on top of that she's delivered about twenty babies a month for nearly two decades. And most importantly, you can go there with her. No topic is off-limits.

My initial response—"Oh my God, really? It's not just me?"—turned to frustration when I realized that we mamas are sorely lacking in a go-to resource for these types of questions. Because I know from previous experiences I had in the years before I started seeing Dr. Bickman, and from conversations with my best girlfriends, that not everyone has such an amazing doctor to sort out the miracle of life for them. My friends who've had babies in the year since I became a mom are constantly asking me these types of questions, too, as if just having a kid is enough to qualify me as a world expert.

I've seen over and over that not every woman has such a cut-and-dried, tell-it-like-it-is obstetrician and experienced mom to dish out sanity-restoring advice at any hour of the day or night. That's why, during a postpartum follow-up one day, Dr. B. and I came up with the idea to write this book.

We wanted to give new moms a go-to place for all the answers they're looking for.

There are so many guides to what our kids need, from the time they're the size of a poppy seed to the time they start kindergarten. But what about what the *mother* needs? It's crazy to watch how quickly our babies' bodies grow, but what about what's happening to *our* bodies? And then we had our big idea. What if we could combine my questions as a new mom with Dr. Bickman's wisdom as a doctor and mother into a go-to book for new mothers?

And that's what we've tried to do in *Whoa, Baby!* I didn't just go to Dr. Bickman for advice, but to my beloved nursing coach for breastfeeding tips. I talked to one of my dear friends, who also happens to be a therapist specializing in postpartum issues, and I spoke with a trainer about working out after baby, and I consulted a physical therapist about the most common recovery issues post-baby. I even talked to a stylist about how to dress in those in-between months when you're done with maternity wear but not quite ready for your skinny jeans.

And throughout it all, we will tell you the whole unvarnished truth. We'll be covering the gross physical stuff (Why does my vagina look like that?); the hormonal and emotional stuff (Why am I crying five times a day when this is the happiest I've ever been?); and the just plain weird stuff (Why did my nipples change color?). We'll be describing scenarios that moms who've already been there and done that will recognize. What happens if I fall asleep with the pump on? Why does sex still hurt when I had a C-section? Why are my legs so swollen? We hope you'll be consulting it before you give birth to prepare you for the messy reality of what's to come, or read it in the middle of the insanity—not that you'll have a chance to read more than a page or two in any given day.

We have all been there. I have, and Dr. B. has, and every single woman who has ever had a baby pulled out of her vagina or abdomen has experienced some version of these changes. But until now, there has never been a place where a new mother could get her down-and-dirty questions answered, except maybe the Internet. And trust me, that is not where you want to turn when you're crouched over a mirror wondering if your vagina will ever return to human dimensions again. Instead, let us hold your hand and walk you through this challenging, bewildering, and wonderful time.

CHAPTER 1

Is There Anything I Can Do to Make This Easier?

(The Final Stretch)

IF YOU'RE ANYTHING LIKE ME, you're used to micromanaging every single little detail of your life. I like to be in charge of my own schedule and my own commitments, and I prefer to do things on my own terms. That was one of the hardest parts of pregnancy for me—just sort of accepting that there was this miracle taking place in my body, and I couldn't really see it or take charge of it. All I could do was let the mysterious creature grow stronger and stronger inside me. And wait and wait and wait.

When I got tired of waiting, I busied myself with what I could control, like getting the house ready. Well, first there was the little matter of moving—when I found out I was pregnant, Tim and I decided to move to a bigger place that would fit our family of three. Moving was a really great excuse to clean out our closets and drawers and just get our lives a bit more organized in anticipation of the Big Change on the horizon. I went into complete nesting overdrive.

And after we settled into the new house, I got totally OCD when it came to prepping for our newest resident! I was going to Restoration Hardware and every other home store in my neighborhood whenever I got a chance. I worked out every last detail of his nursery, making sure every picture I'd chosen for him was hung in the exact right place at the exact right angle. I washed all of his baby clothes and got them all organized in his little closet. I bought crib sheets and one of those breastfeeding pillows, and I set up a nice little diaper-changing station in his room. I even designated a special stretch of the kitchen counter for him, where I could keep all his bottles and pacifiers and a drying rack. I made sure that corner was always extra clean! In short, I was in a complete nesting frenzy those last few months.

Between visits to home stores, I also took care of myself, of course. Most of the time I just felt happy and thrilled for the next chapter in Tim's and my adventure, but on some days I felt really emotional for no apparent reason. I didn't drink caffeine because I thought it made me too excitable, and I tried to do a lot of yoga and work on my breathing whenever I got the chance.

As I got closer to my due date, I made time for the really important preparations, like getting my hair and then eyebrows done—because, hey, if I couldn't control anything that was going on inside my body, at least I could make sure that the outside was looking dope! I got a pedicure, too, even though it felt like it had been months since I'd last been able to see my feet. I just wanted to make myself feel cute since I probably wouldn't be looking all that cute for a while.

With that in mind, I also bought some really luxurious extra-large pajamas and a nightgown with a matching robe that I could wear in the hospital, and some granny underwear. I made up a smooth playlist with songs by Stevie Wonder and the Carpenters. I made a whole list of songs that would relax me and bought several hours' worth (because I believe in buying music) so I could have just the right soundtrack. But beyond that, what else *could* I do?

Toward the end I remember being really calm; it was like I'd finally surrendered to the unknown. Ready or not, that baby was on his way out into the world, and no matter what, I would love him till my dying breath. But as I got bigger and bigger, I started to have more trouble sleeping. Tim would feel me tossing and turning next to him and he'd ask me what was wrong, and I would never have an answer for him. There was nothing wrong at all, beyond some pain in my pelvic region; I was mostly just too excited to sleep.

But despite having the number-one greatest pregnancy of all time, I still had trouble functioning in the morning when I'd spent most of the previous night eating cherry pie and watching the movie *Knocked Up* yet again. I must've watched that movie ten times in the last month of my pregnancy. I'm sure it was because the Katherine Heigl character was pregnant, and when you're pregnant, especially toward the end, you have trouble thinking about anything but pregnancy. That's the only explanation for my other late-night TV-binging obsession, *A Baby Story* on TLC. One night I shrieked out loud because my own Dr. Bickman was in an episode!

As for the rest of it, I tried just to keep on taking those deep breaths and accept that I couldn't stage-manage or choreograph what was about to go down in the delivery room. I asked Dr. Bickman if there was anything I could do to have, or at least come close to, the perfect birth experience, and she laughed and told me there was no such thing. "As long as you and the baby come out on the other end healthy, that's all the perfection you need," she said, and I knew she was right. But again, it's hard, if you're a take-charge personality like me, to let go of the reins.

"A lot of women come to me with questions about what they can do to make the birth process go more smoothly," Dr. Bickman told me. "The honest answer is nothing at all. You've made every doctor's appointment and religiously taken your prenatal vitamins, and now it's entirely out of your hands, which is not what a lot of my Type A patients want to hear."

PRE-BABY CHECKLIST

Whatever you've read, there's nothing you can "do" to get ready for your baby's imminent arrival, but that doesn't mean you won't try! Still, it's important not to overpack, which I'm afraid most of us first-timers do. I confess that I brought concealer and mascara along so I'd be looking my best for the photos! Of course, these remained in my bag the whole time. Here are the preparations that helped me:

- ✔ Pack your hospital bag (but, honestly, all you need is a toothbrush, a change of clothes for the trip home, and your perfect pillow if, like me, you have a favorite. You can bring a cute little onesie for baby, but the hospital will have clothes for the baby, so that's not even necessary. One essential item I wouldn't have known to pack if not for Dr. B.

is socks for the baby: "The hospital will give you clothes and a hat and even mittens, but they won't provide socks, and those can be useful for keeping your baby's tiny feet warm."

- Take a day off. Whether you spend it in the salon (check) or just vegging on the couch in front of your favorite Bravo show, savor every second of quiet time while you can.

- Prepare your house! Make sure you have a place for the baby to sleep, a safe spot for diaper changes, and perhaps most important of all, some comfy spots where you and your loved ones can sit and snuggle the baby, which is the main thing you'll be doing those first few weeks. Maybe stack up some magazines, dig out your remote control, and have some bottles of water handy for the long stretches of sitting ahead of you.

- Relax! Even if it's just for five minutes a day, try to let all your fears— and even all your hopes—go and just relax in the moment. Stay as calm as possible, and the baby inside of you will emerge calm, too.

- Plan on everything deviating from your plans.

Lucky for me, Dr. B. heartily endorsed my pre-baby salon regimen: anything that made me chill out and feel good got the green light from her. "The only thing you can do once you're nearing full term is just try to relax about what's to come," she said. "It's also helpful to take a little time off to pamper yourself, because even if you don't realize it now, you may not get another chance for the next eighteen years. If you've never had a baby before, do something—anything—to indulge yourself, even if it's just taking yourself out for a massage or going to the movies alone in the middle of a weekday. For the first and probably only time in your adult life, you can completely relax with zero guilt. And trust me, this time will not come again, because if you have a second child, you'll still have the first at home to deal with. Taking some time off will also help steel you for the chaos to come."

Dr. Bickman also warned me against getting too hung up on any exact scenario of how the birth was going to go down. I knew that as long as my baby and I ended up healthy, it didn't really matter how we'd gotten there.

"I recently had a patient in labor with her first child after three years—three years!—of trying to get pregnant," Dr. Bickman told me. "But things got a little messy, as they often do when bringing a child into the world. After ninety-five hours—yes, that is almost four days—of labor and three hours of pushing, it became clear that she needed a C-section right away. But she wasn't having it. In between shrieks of agony, she kept screaming, 'I won't do it—this is not what I wanted!'

"I told her it was no longer about what she wanted, it was about the health of the baby, whereupon she burst into tears. 'This is the worst day of my life, this is the worst day of my life,' she kept repeating. I said to her, 'What are you talking about? You're having a baby. This is the best day of your life.' But she kept saying over and over, 'This is a nightmare, this is a nightmare,' and I kept telling her to get a grip: 'This is the opposite of a nightmare. In twenty minutes you're having a baby. Get a grip, get some perspective!' It was only after she finally saw the baby girl she'd wanted for so many years that she finally started to calm down."

I do understand that it's perfectly natural to have some pre-conceived notion of how we want the birth to go; we're only human, after all. But in this one instance, we have to just kind of let it roll. After talking to Dr. B., I went in determined not to freak out about factors totally beyond my control, and I think I did a pretty good job.

"Whether it's your first pregnancy or you've gone through this drill four times already, you probably have some sense of how you want your birth to go," Dr. B. said. "I have patients who walk in and say, 'I want an epidural the instant I have my first contraction,' and I have patients who say, 'No matter what, don't ever give me the option of an epidural.' But we can't al-ways plot out how our labor is going to go. Some of my pa-tients who are convinced they don't want an epidural end up asking for one, and some who do want it don't end up needing one. The whole process of labor is just so unpredictable, and the best approach is just to roll with it. Try, no matter how hard it seems, to just go with the flow."

So if you've never had a baby before, you have no idea what to expect. How do you possibly know what you want? You may have envisioned exactly how it should go, and it's fine to establish a nice foundation of expectations, but above all else you should make flexibility a priority. Dr. Bickman, as well as my amazing doula, told me over and over just to let it happen as it's going to happen, and luckily I got close to my dream sce-nario. And since becoming a mom, I've come to understand that a lot of this new role of mine involves surrendering control of my previous expectations of how things—a dinner out, or a vacation, or even just a trip to the grocery store—are going to be. The adults are no longer completely in the driver's seat, and there's no better time to learn this than during childbirth.

So, I know it's hard, but just trust that your medical providers have your best interests at heart. Your doctor will listen to you and honor your wishes to the greatest degree possible, but the health and safety of the mother and the baby will always come first in their minds—and that's a good thing! "And remember," Dr. Bickman told me, "you're the one we're listening to, not your partner." Tim and I were on the same page about how we wanted the birth to go—we'd communicated nonstop about this in the long weeks leading up to Titan's birth—but apparently that isn't always the case.

"I can't tell you how many times I've walked into a hospital room to find a mom writhing in pain and had the dad look at me and say, 'We're not ready for the epidural yet. We're good,'" Dr. Bickman said. "'We'? Really, 'we'? Whenever this happens, I give the man a look like, 'I didn't ask your opinion, asshole.' Once one of the nurses said to one of these helpful dads, 'Okay, let's take your penis and put it into this door, and then I'll slam the door shut on it every five minutes for thirty-six hours. That's what your wife is going through. Let her answer.'"

(Does everyone understand why I have the best obstetrician in the world?)

So if it's helpful to you, have a talk with your partner about your ideal birth setting, but make sure both of you are on the same page about the countless unforeseen circumstances that can get in the way of that dream scenario. Whatever happens, make sure your partner and you both accept that, like most of the greatest mysteries in life, childbirth can't be planned. After all, it's not a lunch date or a PowerPoint presentation. It's the most incredible miracle you'll ever experience, so just try to surrender control.

CHAPTER 2

Is This Finally Happening for Real?

(The Drama of Delivery)

November 4, 2014: lucky number four. My birthday is on the eleventh and Tim's is on the seventh, so I loved that our family's birthdays all added up. The fourth seemed like the symbolically perfect date to bring Titan into the world.

I checked into the hospital the day before and tried to stay as loose as possible while the inevitable got under way. I catnapped, I ate Popsicles, I had a doula massage my feet, I bounced on one of those big balls and listened to my smooth playlist. I got hooked into my epidural and coasted from there. I wanted my delivery to feel like a party, and it did. We were all singing songs together, trying to serenade the baby out into the world.

Luckily, there was no drama: once Titan was ready to come out, he wasted no time. All of a sudden, I said, "Hey, Doc, there's something really heavy sitting at the bottom of my

> I've delivered something like four thousand babies over the last seventeen years (that's a lot of vaginas!), and they don't always go as smoothly as Kelly's—but again, the only really important thing is that both baby and mother come out healthy, whether you have an "all natural" birth, or a vaginal birth with pain meds, or an induced vaginal birth, or a scheduled C-section, or a C-section after a long labor. How you deliver will likely affect your recovery process, but barring extreme circumstances, it should have no long-term impact on either the baby or you.

vajayjay." Dr. B. picked up the sheet and saw nothing but hair. Four pushes later and he was there! In the end, I delivered in front of not only Tim but also my godmother and two of my godsisters—well, one of them was on FaceTime for the whole experience, but she got to see the whole deal.

After Titan was born, I just did not want him to leave my side—not then or ever again. After waiting and waiting for him to come out for so many months, I was just so excited to meet him! And, because I'd had a pretty easy labor, I wasn't too exhausted to enjoy our brand-new little miracle; it was like I got a second wind when he came out. Luckily, the hospital we'd chosen got me started with skin-to-skin right away, which is what'd I'd wanted. Titan stayed right next to me all day and night, even when the nurses were checking up on him or taking his temperature.

But trust me, I understand exactly how lucky I am, and I know labor doesn't always go that smoothly for everyone. I

have friends who've gone through two whole days of contractions, or who've pushed for six straight hours before having to
get a C-section, and I get that they need a little quiet time to
recover immediately after the baby is born. That's also why it's
so great if you can appreciate and take advantage of everything
the hospital has to offer you. You've got medical experts who
can help you with your every need, and check out your scars,
and take your baby to the nursery if you need a couple of hours
of quiet rest. The hospital is a great place to take the time you
need to start the long process of recovery.

"I always encourage new moms to be with their babies as
much as possible," Dr. Bickman said, "but of course stuff happens, and that's what the nursery is there for. If you need it, use
it! Your baby absolutely won't remember going there, but you
will remember catching up on some much-needed sleep, and
you'll be better prepared to take care of that baby when you're
home from the hospital. And if the baby is in the nursery and
cries, the nurses are going to bring him right back to you—
they're not going to leave the baby crying; they don't want that
either! So do not worry that the baby is going to be crying and
needing you and not getting you. That's just not how it works."

If you've given birth at the hospital, take advantage of everything it offers you. I absolutely loved my time there. I had
Titan by my side, so I was in no hurry to get back to regular
life. That wasn't going to happen anyway, the way my body felt
that week!

"I always have these patients who are in this huge rush to get
back home," Dr. B. said, "and then inevitably—like every single time—they say to me afterward, 'Why was I in such a hurry

to get home?' I hate to say I told you so, but I told you so. I always ask patients, 'What is waiting for you at home that you can't take another twenty-four hours to deal with?' Take your whole four days, or two days if you've had a vaginal birth, or whatever your insurance company will pay for, and make the most of that time to bond with your baby and recover. Sure, you could probably go home the next day if you're an experienced mom and already have four kids at home, but those are the moms who are the most reluctant to leave the hospital, precisely because they know what's waiting for them on the home front! Not everyone has a good support system at home, and pretty soon your partner will go back to work, and it will be just you and the baby and possibly older kids as well. So conserve your energy and take advantage of the hospital to build your energy back up and recover as fast as you can. The time will come when you'll wish you had a parade of nurses coming in and out of your room attending to your every need."

I took Dr. B.'s advice and chilled at the hospital for as long as they'd let me. Sure, my hospital room wasn't exactly the most peaceful place on earth—my whole family was there all day and night, and I had new visitors showing up every twenty or thirty minutes, popping in and out with cafeteria food and causing scenes in the hallway—but that's exactly how I wanted it. I had my precious baby right next to me, I had my husband, and I also had experienced nurses and doctors to help me out if I needed anything.

"And you will have needs, trust me," Dr. Bickman said. "I can't tell you how many patients are surprised by how easy labor seems compared to what comes afterward: the recovery.

So take advantage of everything the hospital has to offer so that you can take care of your body and your baby. Both will need a lot of attention in the coming weeks!"

Yep. Little did I know that my real journey would begin after I left the hospital. Even with my relatively easy labor and delivery, I was still shocked by what happened to my body afterward. The excruciating pain every time I hobbled to the toilet, the HUGE floppy belly, and the days—make that weeks—of bleeding. And I thought pushing Titan's head out was going to be the hardest part! In reality, getting the baby out into the world turned out to be just the beginning of a very long journey back to normal.

CHAPTER 3

Will I Ever Walk Again?

(My Messed-up Lady Parts)

WHEN TITAN FINALLY came out of my body, it was love at first sight. I was so thrilled that my baby boy had come out so healthy and perfect. I honestly could not believe how beautiful he was. I felt like the luckiest woman on earth! But as anyone who's ever given birth knows, that pure rush of joy you feel is always mixed with some other feelings—like pain. You really cannot understand how badly a body can hurt until you have pushed a full-size baby out of such a small opening. The second the adrenaline from the labor had worn off and I'd accomplished my goal of getting that baby out into the world, I immediately became aware of an excruciating pain in my nether regions.

And, yes, even as I was gazing for the first time at my gorgeous miracle of a son, I was beginning to feel a little concerned about how much my vajayjay hurt. Okay, "concerned" is an understatement. I was full-on panicking. What had happened down there? How could my vagina hurt so bad? And why was it all loose and floppy—would it always be like this? Could the doctor sew it up so it would be tight again? And what could it possibly look like—was it ever going to be cute again? Was my husband ever going to want to enter back in there again? Forget that—would I ever be able to walk normally again? What if I had to undergo vaginal surgery? What was vaginal surgery, anyway? Could it possibly hurt more than what I'd just gone through?

So, yes, in spite of my total happiness, every single one of these thoughts flashed through my brain in the three minutes after I pushed Titan out. Because, man, my vagina hurt. What had I ever done to deserve this? It seriously felt like an open wound that just ached and burned and ached and throbbed. I couldn't turn over in my hospital bed without feeling like my whole body was going to be ripped open right at my center. I'd torn a lot on my left side and I could not imagine ever feeling like myself again. Dr. Bickman came by my room to check on me, and I was practically in tears. "What happened to me?" I asked her. "Why does it still hurt so bad? Did I do something wrong?"

Once again, she immediately talked me down. "Listen, you might not hear about it in those cheerful weekly emails you get from the baby website, but almost every single first-timer giving birth vaginally tears."

I shook my head in disbelief. There was no way that all the other mothers out there had experienced this type of intense vaginal pain. Otherwise the world would be filled with only-children because why would a woman willingly put herself through that torture again once she already knew what she was in for? And why hadn't my friends who were already moms told me just how bad it would hurt?

"Roughly 95 percent of first-time moms have some form of tear," Dr. Bickman told me. "And if you think about it, it's the 5 percent who don't tear who are the weird ones! Getting a baby out of your body is like trying to shove a bowling ball through a pinhole. Something's gotta give, and guess what? It's not going to be the bowling ball. The softer thing loses, and that's the opening to your vagina. It's inevitable that you're going to tear."

I only had second-degree tearing and I still couldn't sit down for three weeks—I was so angry about it! I couldn't imagine what women who've had it worse have had to endure. The female body truly has gone through it all and then some when it comes to the business of birthing babies.

But still—because this is just the way I think—I did wonder if I could've prevented the tearing, if I should've somehow prepared my body for the trauma beforehand. Were there exercises I should've been practicing or products I should've been buying to keep my vagina in one piece? Should I have asked my trainer to get me on some supersonic vaginal training regimen before the big event? I am a can-do kind of girl, so I like to do my part when possible.

Here again Dr. Bickman set me straight, telling me that there was really nothing I could've done to prevent tearing. "Don't beat yourself up about it—your body is already beaten up enough as it is," she said. "Some patients try to prepare by doing massage and applying special oils, but the truth of the matter is that in that moment the baby's head is putting the

TYPES OF TEARS

Ninety-five percent of first-time mothers tear somewhere with their first baby, but not all of them tear in the same place. It's possible to tear anywhere in that region, but the most common type is right down the midline. That type of tear is broken into four categories:

First degree. This is the lightest type of tear, and it's really more like a skid mark than an actual abrasion. None of the muscles are affected at all, just tissue. If it didn't bleed, your doctor almost wouldn't have to sew it up at all, but because that tissue is so vascular—that is, filled with a ton of blood vessels—even the most superficial abrasion will bleed. A Band-Aid would almost be sufficient to control it, but you obviously can't put a Band-Aid down there, so we stitch it up and it disappears before you know it.

Second degree. This is the next-deepest level of tear, which goes to the muscle and needs suturing. While these tears can be painful for several weeks, they usually heal with no complications, and they're certainly incredibly common. I would say that roughly 80 percent of women experience this type of tear on delivering their first baby.

Third and fourth degree. Only an estimated 4 percent of women have these far more serious lacerations, which go deep into the muscle. Fourth-degree tears can be particularly brutal, going all the way down to the anus, and might even require surgery later on to

pressure on your vagina, and some ripping is almost certainly going to occur. But don't worry, because in the vast majority of cases your vagina will heal, no surgery necessary."

I had a lot of trouble believing her in those days when I could hardly sit down on a wooden chair without letting out a shriek correct, but luckily they are very, very rare. I honestly can't remember the last fourth-degree laceration I've had to repair.

You can tear in all sorts of other places as well—really anything goes when it comes to childbirth. You can tear on the top of your vagina, and you can also tear your labia, which is very easy to fix but can be painful since it's on the outside and patients can feel the urine running over the cuts when they pee. Patients with labial tears often call me complaining that they have a bladder infection, but it's really just the urine irritating the cuts. It's like when you bite your lip and it bleeds a lot but then goes away quickly—it's the same kind of tissue there. If we didn't sew it up, it would heal on its own, but sewing definitely speeds up the process. The outside tearing we sew up because it cuts back on the bleeding and will look better in the long run.

You might also be coping with what's called an episiotomy, which is an incision made by the doctor to speed up delivery. Doctors usually make this cut when the fetus is in distress of some sort or the mother is too exhausted to continue pushing; some women have a tight tissue that needs to be cut because it prevents the vagina from stretching enough for the baby's head to come out. While I myself do episiotomies rarely, other doctors do them as a standard delivery procedure. An episiotomy is about the equivalent of a second-degree tear in terms of discomfort, and it heals exactly the same way.

of pain. Was that it then? Had giving birth actually ruined my vaj for life? Sure, Dr. Bickman had seen quite a few cooters in her day, but I had trouble believing that other women had it as bad as me down there. While these anxieties were running through my head, I made the mistake of getting out a mirror and trying to study the situation. Talk about the world's worst idea! When I finally caught a glimpse of the orifice that was causing me so much pain and sorrow, I almost screamed out loud. That bloody battlefield was my vagina? Was it going to look like that forever? Would Tim ever want to come near that nasty scene again? Not that I'd blame him if he didn't, given what I'd just seen.

I know Dr. Bickman had already tried to calm me down, but I couldn't help but ask her again. Titan was almost a month old at this point, but from the look of my vagina, I'd only just pushed him out an hour earlier. If this is what she meant by "healing," then we were working with some seriously different definitions of the term.

But again, Dr. B. was prepared for my freak-out. When I brought this fear to her, she smiled, because this, too, she had heard quite a few times before. She told me that the only problem was that I'd tried to inspect my raw, swollen vagina. "Of course it looks terrible!" she told me. "You would not believe the number of patients I've had who've gotten their husbands to take pictures of their vaginas when they've been home from the hospital all of thirty minutes—I can only say, no! Gross! Just stop it!

"Just last week," Dr. Bickman said, "a patient showed up at my office when her baby was three days old. Before I could ask her what was wrong, she whipped out her cell phone and pushed it across my desk, treating me to an extremely vivid close-up photograph of her vagina. 'Look at it!' she cried. 'Have you ever seen anything so awful?'"

Dr. Bickman went on: "I immediately gave her back her phone and said, 'What are you even doing taking a camera down there? I don't go down there with a camera on a good day—or make that ever! Why are you taking pictures of your vagina seventy-two hours after you pushed out a baby? Of course it looks disgusting: you just pushed out a baby!' But the patient wasn't having it. She kept saying, 'No, no, but there's something wrong with it. What do I do? It looks infected!' Infected—do you know how many women have used that word to describe their postpartum vaginas? Over and over I've had to say, 'Yes, it's not so attractive down there right now, but that doesn't mean it's infected. That's just what a vagina looks like right after giving birth.'" (I have to admit that I had briefly wondered about an infection myself. But while infections do happen, they are relatively rare.)

"Again, think about the size of your vagina and the size of your newborn baby—there's not a vagina in the world that's not going to be altered by those acrobatics. In the weeks after birth, your vagina is not meant to be examined by anyone except a medical professional, who can react to it properly," Dr. Bickman told me.

So I am going to repeat her advice and tell you to do yourself (and your doctor!) a favor and just stay out of there right after childbirth. Put away the selfie stick. Do not look in that region when you've just come home from the hospital, and definitely don't capture the image on your cell phone for posterity. Just leave your vagina alone! Keep it clean and otherwise just stay away. It will heal like it's supposed to, and if it doesn't, then your doctor will let you know at your postpartum visit and you can go from there. In the meantime, you're not doing anyone any favors with that cell-phone camera. Save it for snaps of your baby's adorable mug.

GETTING THE GEAR

Let someone else deal with the diapers. Don't leave the hospital without all the gear you need! The first twenty-four hours, you get to enjoy (well, that's not quite the right word) these maxi pads that double as ice packs. After that, you can wear pads that double as vagina warmers—sounds crazy, but you will really want to load up on these guys, as they provide a lot of relief. Make sure you have your pain meds and your stool softener handy, and don't forget to grab that sitz bath for soaking several times a day, and one of those squirt bottles so you can hose yourself down every time you pee. I'd also recommend one of those donuts for making sitting on the toilet a little less excruciating those first few days. And grab as many pairs of those mesh underwear as the nurses will allow!

CHAPTER 4

Why Didn't Anybody Tell Me to Bring Depends?

(Postpartum Bleeding)

ONE OF THE BEST THINGS about being pregnant is that you get a break from your monthly periods. Yeah, your body is getting large and in charge and, even in the best of pregnancies, you're more tired than usual and you have occasional heartburn and you can't walk up a flight of stairs without panting, but, hey— at least you don't have to worry about tossing tampons in your purse! But then, once you give birth, you might be surprised by how the blood flow from your uterus returns with a vengeance. That little wriggling baby is just the beginning of what you'll be ejecting from your body in those first few weeks.

I literally had no idea how much I was going to bleed after I gave birth. Just no clue. It was like getting five periods at once. Seriously, the after-birth bleeding experience was like the heavy-flow day of my period jacked up to eleven. The bleeding seemed to go on forever, too, and whenever I walked I had this uncomfortable chafing sensation between my legs. But, hey, at least it wasn't my period, right?

"Postpartum bleeding is definitely not your period if you're breastfeeding," Dr. Bickman said. "It's just your womb emptying itself out of all the blood and gunk that's been surrounding your baby for the duration of your pregnancy, and the amount varies a lot from woman to woman. Some women who've had C-sections hardly bleed afterward; others bleed for weeks." I was definitely in the bleeding-for-weeks category.

Okay, so the bleeding was normal and not my time of the month; that was a relief. But why was there so damn much blood? Where was it coming from and how could my body possibly hold so much of it? Hadn't carrying a big baby around been enough?

Once again Dr. B. set me straight, reminding me that my blood volume had increased by roughly 50 percent during my pregnancy, which is why my gums seemed to be hemorrhaging when I went to the dentist for a standard teeth-cleaning during my second trimester. "When your pregnancy is over," Dr. Bickman said, "your body is now getting rid of the excess fluids. You'll also be shedding a lot of a mucusy substance known as lochia, which is an appetizing combination of blood, bacteria, and uterine tissue. This whole process can last up to six weeks." So just like everything else that seemed so topsy-turvy, all that blood and gunk streaming out of my body was totally part of the whole postpartum package. Nice.

My next challenge was figuring out how to manage the blood flow without ruining all the lovely nightgowns I'd purchased for my dream birthing experience. Obviously tampons

QUICK FACTS ABOUT POSTPARTUM BLEEDING

- It's not your period: you're shedding what's called lochia, a combination of blood, mucus, and uterine tissue. You might also be shedding your stitches and sutures, which kind of form into a scab inside your vagina, in the discharge.

- Remember how your blood volume doubled during pregnancy? Most of this bleeding is just your body getting itself back to normal blood levels.

- Do not use tampons until after your six-week checkup. You don't want to be bringing any new bacteria into that part of your body right now!

- The bleeding should decrease a little every day after birth. If it doesn't, consult a medical professional.

- This bleeding should last a total of four to six weeks.

---

were out of the question for the possibility of introducing bad bacteria into my body, not that I had any desire to introduce a foreign object to that region of my body after it had gone through so much already! (The same went for sex in those tender early days; sorry about that, Tim.)

Instead I relied on that dope disposable Ace bandage underwear they gave me at the hospital because, trust me, you are not going to want to wear your sexy lingerie when you're in a hospital bed with a big-ass stomach and a bloody vagina. I also became totally dependent on these monster maxi pads that came with my postpartum kit and fit nicely inside my gigantic granny undies, even if, that first week, they weren't nearly strong enough for me. I had to change them all the time—like, we are talking every hour. Early on, it seemed like as soon as I put a new pad on, it'd be soaked through and I'd have to grab a replacement. If I wasn't working on breastfeeding Titan, I was swapping out my underwear or changing my sheets.

Next time, I am definitely going to stockpile both the mesh underwear and those pads so I can rock them for the whole month after I get home from the hospital without having to send Tim out on emergency drugstore runs. Or I may take it to the next level and go for some protection that goes all the way around me, like Depends. Now that is what I wish I'd had after Titan! If the baby gets diapers, why don't I? For the full 360-degree protection, you heard it here first. You need to get yourself some Depends. I'm loading up for my next baby.

"But be warned that wearing pads all the time—not that you have a choice—can cause some serious irritation," Dr. Bickman said. "The pad traps in moisture, which is the whole point of it, of course, and that can get uncomfortable. A lot of women get yeast infections postpartum, but that has as much to do with being on antibiotics and having roller-coaster hormones than the pads." So keep those sitz baths going around the clock to keep that area maximally clean and fresh . . . well, as "fresh" as your vagina can possibly be after going through such a trauma!

Basically, unless you're in the market for new linens and even a new mattress, you don't really have a choice those first weeks, so you'd best learn to love those pads. And like so much of this crazy phase, you'll stop bleeding once you've really convinced yourself that it's going to go on forever. The problem for me was that right when the postpartum bleeding stopped, the regular period bleeding started. Everyone told me that as long as I was breastfeeding, I wouldn't have my period, and I have to admit that I was excited—but nope, I got my period pretty much right away, with no break.

"Look at it this way," Dr. Bickman said, "it's a good sign of ovarian function! Statistically, 85 percent of moms won't get their period while breastfeeding. Of the other 15 percent, it could be one month, or it could be three months. It's just totally random. After six to eight weeks, you shouldn't have any more of that stuff coming out of your body, but before six to eight weeks it's almost impossible for your ovaries to have ovulated, and once you do get it you may not get it every month. If you go away on a vacation and you're feeding baby more formula, you may ovulate. But then, when you get home, you may go back to feeding more and your ovaries might get suppressed again and so your period might not come on schedule the next time. Until you're totally done breastfeeding, it could be regular or irregular—there's just no set pattern that you can rely on. The same is true of when you are able to get pregnant again; it's totally different with every kid. After my first kid, I got pregnant again without ever having had my period. After my fifth kid, I got my period three months after giving birth. There is absolutely no way to predict it in advance!"

After the weeks of nonstop bleeding, getting my regular old period again was almost a relief. I'd never complain about it again! Well, almost never.

CHAPTER 5

Has Anyone Ever Been This Heavy?

(Swelling and Sweating)

YOU KNOW HOW you always get really bloated the couple of days before your period, and the clothes that fit you the previous evening now barely zip up? (Or maybe that's just me.) Well, there's that normal kind of PMSy bloated, and then there's being so bloated that your body seems to have lost all shape. In the weeks after having Titan, I fell firmly in category two. Even a few months later, when I was leaving the house more regularly, I'd try out those little waist cinchers, but I still felt like an inflatable toy, like someone had literally blown air directly into my body.

I will never forget the first time I got up out of my hospital bed after giving birth. As I dragged myself across the room, I couldn't believe how heavy I felt! A big human baby had just exited my body, so why did I feel even more pregnant than I had when I was carrying him in my belly? I was completely puffy and my stomach seemed even bigger than it had the previous day, when it was packed to the gills with a baby.

GETTING YOUR WEDDING RING OFF

By the end of my third trimester, my wedding ring didn't come close to fitting—it looked like a corset wrapped tightly around my finger—so I took it off. It was that or saw it off my finger if I'd waited a couple more days. "I tell people to get a new ring," Dr. Bickman said. "More diamonds—and you'd better buy them now, because you won't have any money later. Or, for a cheaper solution, you can also try some Preparation H on your finger. It's a steroid cream, and the steroids are an anti-inflammatory that make your skin shrink a little, which helps your ring slide off better." Three cheers to the mamas who wear their rings till the bitter end of pregnancy. I have friends whose fingers are swollen but they just aren't bothered by that tight ring. I couldn't stand it; I was afraid I'd have to saw it off my finger if I waited another day!

And, even weirder, I couldn't stop sweating. From that very first day and for weeks afterward, I had sweat dripping out of every pore—and it smelled nasty, too, a very specific, peculiar smell I have never encountered before or since. Dr. Bickman told me that this was all part of the program: "You'll wake up drenched and wind up changing clothes five times a day (and not just from baby spit-up), yet another symptom that causes some patients to call me in a panic. I get phone calls all the time with patients saying, 'I can't stop sweating, Dr. Bickman, I think I have an infection. I need to go to the ER!'

"Before the total panic sets in, I'll first try to identify the source of the infection. Where are you sweating from? Is it your back? Is it your nipples? Is it your kidneys? The answer is almost always no, no, no. And that's because in the

vast majority of cases there is no infection. You're sweating because, when you breastfeed, you're suppressing your ovaries
and not ovulating, and as a consequence your estrogen takes
a nosedive. Just look up the classic symptoms of menopause,
also associated with a sharp drop in estrogen, and you'll see
the same symptoms: the hot flashes, the out-of-control body
temperature, the constant sweating. The cause is usually not
an infectious fever; it's probably just a resetting of your internal thermostat from the hormonal changes your body is going
through. As for the distinctive smell, which always overpowers
me when I walk into a hospital recovery room, that comes from
a combination of sweat and hormones. I think it's just nature's
way of telling your husband to stay away from you until you've
been cleared for sexual activity again."

My internal temperature was completely out of whack—
one minute I'd be freezing to death and the next I'd feel like
I was about to pass out from heatstroke—and still the sweat
kept on pouring out of me. I just got into the habit of changing
my clothes almost as often as the baby's and sometimes even
sleeping on top of a towel (which would always be soaking wet
when I got up). Luckily, I stopped sweating so much after the
first two weeks, but I couldn't shake that inflatable-doll feeling.
What was happening to my body and when would it stop?

"You get tons of fluid through an IV in labor," Dr. Bickman told me, "and after you have the baby, you still have all
the fluid in your blood vessels that you've been pumping into
your veins. Your capillaries will get leaky and the blood will
migrate into your tissue, and from there it takes a few weeks
for that fluid in your tissue to go back into your bloodstream

when you can pee it out. It takes your kidneys a long time to process all of that pee! In the meantime, it's totally par for the course for people to feel bloated. I get calls all the time, a week out, from people saying, 'I'm so bloated! Something happened—what's wrong with me?' And I always have to reassure them that 'No, no, nothing's wrong; it's just the fluid coming out of your blood vessels into your tissue,' but it still takes some time to pee it out gradually. Unlike a lot of postpartum symptoms, the bloating is often worse on days seven through ten when the moms have already left the hospital and gone back home."

All the nurses and doctors in the hospital kept telling me to drink more and more fluids, which at first felt really counterintuitive to me, because I felt like my body couldn't possibly contain any more liquid, not to mention that I was leaking urine like crazy in those days. But I like to stick to the program, so I started drinking tons, just tons, of water, and I did feel like it was helping to cleanse my body. By the end of the first month, I felt (and looked, I hope!) a good deal less bloated, and I kept on chugging down huge quantities of water every day.

Still, for weeks afterward, my fingers, stomach, and face remained super puffy. It turns out that this reaction, what's known as edema, is a very common side effect of giving birth. There's a lot of progesterone that builds up in your body during pregnancy, and that can make you retain more water and swell up. Those levels don't necessarily drop right away. Also, if you're hooked up to an IV during delivery, fluids can accumulate in your body very quickly and, as Dr. B. explained, take weeks to depart it.

HOW TO REDUCE THE BLOAT

- ✔ Ditch the processed food or any of your go-tos that have a high sodium content. Salt will make you retain water longer.

- ✔ Eat a high-fiber diet heavy on the fresh fruits and vegetables.

- ✔ You just can't drink enough water! Even if it feels like you're making the problem worse, more water will mean less water retention in the long run.

You will find yourself peeing all the time, and that's a good thing! Just as with the sweating, your body is working to get rid of excess fluid, either through your pores or through your bladder. You will be peeing constantly and sweating like a pig. Just learn to love it, because the more you flush out now, the sooner you'll be back to normal (the new normal, that is).

But that wasn't my only difficulty. Just as I was done worrying about the bloat, I had another concern: a slight tingling at the tips of my fingers and toes. What was up with that?

Dr. Bickman told me that this was just another side effect of the swelling. All that swelling presses on your nerves, and the ones you feel the most are the farthest from your heart, like the tips of your toes and your fingertips, which can lead to numbness. Your bigger-than-usual uterus can block the blood flowing elsewhere in your body, which can also cause you to feel numb at your extremities. When you're pushing, your body relays extra blood to hands and feet. All of these things can cause numbness after birth, and it can last as long as three months.

"People call me all the time saying, 'I have MS! I have carpal tunnel! I need to see a specialist!'" Dr. Bickman told me. "So I ask, 'Is the swelling on both sides?' and they say yes. I then ask, 'Is it worse in the morning?' Again they say yes. Both of those things are a sign that this is normal post-pregnancy swelling and will subside just as you've had a chance to freak out about it. That doesn't mean it's much fun while it lasts. But as the swelling all over your body goes down, so do the pressure and the numbness."

Other tricks that helped me with the swelling situation in those first few weeks: I tried not to stand up for too long at any one time, which wasn't that hard since I'd just given birth and was either breastfeeding or trying to get sleep pretty much around the clock. I also kept my legs at a slight upward angle to get the blood moving down from my feet more. Reflexology was also great for me—and I loved getting foot rubs from Tim whenever he wasn't too busy cooing over the baby!

CHAPTER 6

Will I Ever Be Able to Go #2 Again?

(Constipation)

ONCE YOU'VE pushed out an entire human baby, you should have no trouble pushing out a little poop, right? Oh, if only life were so simple. I was totally, perhaps irrationally, freaked out by the prospect of going #2 after giving birth. Since I'd torn down there, I had all sorts of worst-case scenarios floating through my mind at all hours of the night and day. What if the doc hadn't stitched me up right? What if pooing messed up my stitches and I tore all over again? What if when I tried to poo it came out the wrong hole?

I'd read all about fistulas, where the tissue between the rectum and the vagina breaks down, and I knew how horrible they could be for women in countries with less advanced medical care. Sure, it was probably crazy for me, who had given birth in one of the best hospitals in the richest country in the world, to worry about those potential catastrophes, but if you've ever gone three days without sleep while trying to take care of a newborn and learn how to breastfeed, you'll know just where I'm coming from mentally.

And physically, of course, I really, really needed to go. I was so stuffed up that first week—I felt like I was carrying another whole baby in there!—but it didn't feel like anything was going to emerge on its own. Since I'd torn pretty bad on my left side, I had trouble even just sitting on the toilet in the weeks after delivery. I wish someone had told me about those donut cushions that you can rig up underneath you to relieve the pressure. Those would've helped me a lot, just in terms of allowing me to lower myself onto the toilet with a relative degree of comfort.

But, meanwhile, the hours were ticking by and I was still seeing no action in that department. Titan was pooing a lot— why couldn't I? It wasn't as if all sorts of other substances weren't coming out of my body. I was bleeding like crazy and peeing what felt like every ten minutes—sometimes a trickle directly in my Ace-bandage underwear when I couldn't get to the bathroom in time—but #2 just wasn't happening. And the more constipated I felt, the more worried I got; the more time that elapsed, the more scared I got that having my first post-partum bowel movement would be as painful as delivering a seven-and-a-half-pound baby.

So what did I do? You guessed it. I called Dr. Bickman. She immediately calmed me down and told me that, contrary to popular belief, she got more panic-stricken calls about con-stipation than about vaginal issues. She offered a whole list of reasons women like me could get constipated after pregnancy. I could relate to several of them.

- You had a long labor and went a few days without food.
- Your rectum lost some muscle power from all the pushing.
- You're unconsciously holding it in because you fear more pain in that region.
- Your prenatal vitamin—and, if you're taking it, iron as well—could be contributing to the blockage.
- The anti-nausea meds some women are prescribed might also be a culprit.
- The painkillers you're taking to recover from childbirth are probably clogging you up most of all.

This last one surprised me. I hadn't known that the prescription painkillers I took those first three days for the unbelievable pain in my vajayjay could've been clogging up my digestion. Dr. Bickman told me that I should absolutely keep taking them—ditto for my prenatal vitamins—but I just had to be aware of what they were doing to my body and make a few adjustments. And every time I did take them, I also needed to be taking a stool softener to counteract their constipating effects. "Worst-case scenario, you get a little diarrhea," Dr. Bickman said. "Isn't that better than extreme constipation?" I couldn't argue with that. But in addition to taking stool softeners, I also had to get over my mental fear of letting go, so to speak.

"The longer you hold it in, the worse it will be," Dr. Bickman told me. "If you're worried that pushing out some poo now will hurt, just think how bad it will be if you wait three more days. I promise you do not want to go there. Unless you are squeezing out the most gigantic dinosaur turd in the world, your vaginal stitches will be fine with a little pushing—and the same goes for C-section stitches. Anyway, that whole region of your body will probably be pretty numb those first few days, so the process will likely end up less painful than you think if you get it over with as early as possible. Holding it in might make other aspects of your recovery worse, too, since constipation can be a strain to the pelvic floor. Also, if you already have hemorrhoids (more on that in the next chapter), the strain of an extremely hard bowel movement could exacerbate the problem."

To make sure I was doing everything I could, I also upped the fiber intake of my diet (within reason, of course, since I didn't want to eat raw food that might give Titan gas while I was breastfeeding), and that ended up helping with my fluid retention, too. I avoided white bread and other constipating foods while drinking tons and tons of water—turns out that drinking a lot is not only good for bloating, but for bowel movements, too. A good thing, because if you're breastfeeding, you'll feel insanely dehydrated around the clock anyway.

I also tried to move around as much as I could. I don't mean go-to-the-gym moving, but more like get-out-of-bed-and-pace-the-room moving, which was about all I could handle at that point. Some regular light motion, like walking down the block, helped not just my bowels, but my whole body.

Last but not least, I saw a reflexologist who rubbed everything out, or at least she helped me feel more relaxed about the necessity of doing the deed; she also helped with my bloating. Once I finally went through with it, I came to understand that a lot of what was holding me back was just psychological! After giving birth to Titan, I felt like I'd done enough pushing for a lifetime, and I wasn't ready to go down that path again just yet. Getting a nice rubdown helped me chill for a bit and be less anxious.

And guess what? After a few more days, everything finally went back to its regularly scheduled programming. (I'll spare you any more details, but let's just say it wasn't nearly as excruciating as I thought.)

**Recommended High-Fiber Foods
(That Also Happen to Be Good for Breastfeeding)**

Water, water, and more water
Raspberries, apples, and pears
Raisins, prunes, and other old-lady foods
Brown rice, quinoa, and oatmeal
Lentils, split peas, black beans, lima beans, chickpeas
Artichokes, broccoli, peas, squash
Avocados
Flax and chia seeds

CHAPTER 7

What Are These Bumps on My Butt?

(Hemorrhoids)

DR. BICKMAN HAD already told me that constipation was probably the most common reason she got panicked phone calls after normal deliveries. But guess what else is high on the list? Hemorrhoids, which turn out to be an incredibly common side effect of childbirth. Of course, knowing how many women get them (a lot) doesn't make it any less scary when you suddenly discover your butt is covered all over in bumps. I speak from experience, and I'll confess here and now that I dealt with this unpleasant surprise for an entire year after Titan was born. It's hard to talk about hemorrhoids because, well, they're completely disgusting, but when I understood the very normal mechanisms that caused them to pop up, so to speak, I felt somewhat reassured. (But that sure doesn't mean I was eager to talk about them with Tim in the room.)

"Hemorrhoids are basically like varicose veins on your ass," Dr. Bickman told me. "It's the exact same physiology, the result of too much pressure on your veins." She explained in detail how you wake up one day with these unappetizing bumps on your butt.

Contributing Factor 1: Your veins are working too hard.

Arteries actively pump blood from the heart, but veins, which send blood back to the heart, are much more passive—they just kind of kick back and let the blood do all the work. They're equipped with these little valves designed to push the blood back up to your heart, but in pregnancy your blood volume almost doubles, so those little valves often get overworked and overwhelmed trying to get all that blood back to your heart. Add to that the growing size of your uterus, which is putting pressure on the veins of your pelvis and causing them to become inflamed.

Contributing Factor 2: Your uterus is too big.

Your large-and-in-charge uterus is pushing down on your butt like a gigantic watermelon, which causes the blood flow through your veins to slow down and the veins on your butt to swell up. (I know, such an attractive image, right?) As your uterus shrinks back to normal dimensions in the six weeks after childbirth, the evidence of strain-on-your-butt veins should subside as well.

> ### OTHER HEMORRHOID-LIKE SURPRISES
>
> Some women also get varicose veins on the lips of their vagina, which can really cause them to panic, and no wonder, because it looks like a third vulva sticking out. As with so much else, I don't bring up this less-than-attractive side effect of pregnancy unless the woman asks. ("Out of sight, out of mind" is a helpful motto for those first few weeks postpartum.) In most cases, the hemorrhoids will go away on their own within the first six weeks, and their unpleasantness will fade from your mind … until your next pregnancy!

Contributing Factor 3: You're constipated.

For all the reasons we discussed in the last chapter (taking iron, prenatal vitamins, painkillers, and so on), you're having more trouble than usual doing the deed (no, not that deed— that's still off the table for now) in the weeks after having a kid. There's an abundance of progesterone in your body during pregnancy, which can make your veins relax and make you even more constipated. And when you're constipated, you have to push harder to get a bowel movement into the world, which puts even more pressure on your veins and makes your hemorrhoids get even gnarlier. This is another big reason why it's so important to keep your digestive system running on time: you don't want those hemorrhoids to bleed when you're trying to go to the bathroom. To get rid of them, you need to be able to go to the bathroom without too much straining.

Contributing Factor 4: You just pushed out a big baby!

Talk about overworked veins! The intense physical pressure of pushing that baby out into the world in the final stages of labor can really cause those hemorrhoids to explode into overdrive, which is why hemorrhoids are more common after vaginal births (though definitely also possible after a C-section). Your poor exhausted veins bulge out and become twisted and enlarged.

Dr. Bickman also told me that I might've had hemorrhoids during my pregnancy but I just didn't notice them till after the fact. "In the last weeks of pregnancy, you have so many other physical complaints that the hemorrhoids just have to take their place in line. And it's not like, with your big stomach in the way, you can just peer down and give yourself an exam." Even if I'd acquired my hemorrhoids during labor, it's possible that I wouldn't have noticed them right away, either, both because I had a lot of other stuff going on at that particular moment and because the epidural (and subsequent pain meds I got for my tearing) was keeping the pain at bay.

"It's usually not until women have been home from the hospital for a few days that I get a phone call with a shriek of 'What is this on my ass?'" Dr. Bickman said, pretty much recounting exactly the phone call I had placed to her when I noticed the gnarly new additions down there.

RELIEVING HEMORRHOIDS

Cortisone cream. Some doctors prescribe a steroid cream to help with the pain—and, no, it won't hurt the baby.

Ice packs. Don't be afraid to stick that ice right where it hurts! No one's looking, so go for it. You can also get those dope disposable ice packs that you wear in your underwear like a maxi pad. These can be very helpful those first few days.

Sitz bath. Soaking your butt in a warm sitz bath will help heal the birth site and also encourage your hemorrhoids to shrink.

Squirt bottle. Every time you have a bowel movement, squirt that whole region of your body to make sure everything is squeaky clean down there.

Tucks wipes. These witch-hazel wipes can provide much-needed 'rhoids relief.

Tylenol or Advil. If your hemorrhoids are still bothering you after you've recovered from other painful aspects of childbirth, you can take over-the-counter painkillers a few times a day to relieve the pain.

As with so many of these delightful post-baby developments, the hemorrhoids should go away on their own. If they decide to stick around for what seems like far too long, talk to your doctor to make sure everything's okay. In the early days, you can't do much more than try to keep as regular as possible, because the stress of pushing out rock-hard poos can injure your body all over again.

CHAPTER 8

Will I Ever Sleep Again?

(The New Nighttime Schedule)

WHEN TITAN WAS a couple of weeks old, I had some good friends from out of town come over to snuggle him. I was so excited to show off my baby boy, I'd been looking forward to seeing them all day. But when we all settled on the couch together, everyone was chatting and my girlfriend was cooing over Titan and all of a sudden, I was just out. Completely unconscious midway through a conversation while sitting upright on the couch.

After I don't know how long, I heard laughter in the background and I opened my eyes and realized that my mouth had been hanging wide open and there was this huge string of drool dripping down my chest. "Sorry about that—where were we?" I tried to rejoin the conversation, but I was too far gone by that point. My friend gave me a little hug and said, "Kelly, just go to bed. We've got the baby, there's milk in the fridge—just go have a nap and please let us take care of Titan!"

I was such a zombie at this point that I just grunted, "Huh?" and felt myself being led out of the room. I had zero idea what was going on, and when I finally woke up, my friends were long gone, but I felt clearheaded for the first time in weeks. I had really, really, really needed that sleep.

As every mother learns, sleep deprivation is an incredibly powerful force, and a *huge* part of what makes new motherhood such a challenge for those of us accustomed to getting our eight hours of shut-eye every night. If you're not getting enough sleep (and in those early days I was getting almost none), it is impossible to think straight or eat right or take care of your baby. Forget catching up with an old friend you haven't seen in a year! If you're not sleeping, it is just game off.

Of course, in many ways I had it easier than most people, since I had a ton of help from Tim and my family, not to mention that we splurged on a baby nurse during the first several weeks Titan was home from the hospital, which I still believe is the best money I've ever spent in my entire life. But even with all those extra sets of hands, I still always had one eye open and one eye closed.

One reason is that I was totally committed to breastfeeding and, since I was the only one who could handle that aspect of baby-rearing, I made sure I got up whenever Titan was hungry, which was, unfortunately, every ninety minutes. Yep, I didn't have one of those newborns who slurped his fill and then snoozed for half the night; I had one of those newborns who wanted to start his next feeding what felt like minutes after he'd finished his last one.

For the first five days after we got home, I thought, "I got this," but after that I crashed—hard. When it came time to breastfeed him at 11:00, 12:30, 2:00, 3:30 . . . I started to feel like I just couldn't do it. When you're completely and totally exhausted, you lose all perspective on, well, everything.

By the end of the second week, as I drowsed through several post-midnight feedings, I'd feel like my arms were barely strong enough to hold him, and I was terrified that I would drop him while he was at the boob, or even worse, fall asleep right on top of him. I was trying to be up when he was up and ready when he was ready, but I was so tired that I became worried my body wasn't producing as much milk as it should, and that added to the stress my utter fatigue was causing.

The act of breastfeeding itself was physically draining to me as well. On some of those nights, it felt like Titan was sucking the energy out of me with every drop of milk. And my fears weren't entirely ungrounded, for another time while I was in the middle of breastfeeding, Tim started shaking me, crying, "The baby, the baby!" because I'd dropped off for a split second while holding him on me.

Every mom has her own strategies for powering though this fatigue, and I asked Dr. Bickman how she managed to endure this sleep deprivation five times—I just couldn't imagine!— while, being the ultimate badass that she is, going back into work mere days after giving birth. She, of course, had some amazing suggestions.

Sleep Rule 1: Stay in bed as long as you can.

"I never had a baby nurse, but I did have a rule. I didn't want my feet to touch the floor all night," Dr. Bickman said. "For all five of our babies, my husband and I worked out a nice division of labor. I would stay in bed and feed the baby—I was the only one who could, after all—and he would have to do everything else. He could get the diaper and the wipes and change the clothes and tighten the swaddle and whatever else needed doing. I would be in charge of just the feeding, and that was a lot. I found that minimizing what I needed to do helped me focus both on the baby and on my own needs. The flip side of that is that the baby often stayed in bed with me, since it was easier for me simply to roll over and start the feeding. That was the only way I could get enough sleep to show up at work the next day. Of course, when my kids got older it was much harder to kick them out."

Sleep Rule 2: Don't be afraid to accept help.

This doesn't apply just to sleep, but to all sorts of aspects of life post-pregnancy. Whatever path you choose, accept whatever help that's offered you whenever you can: say yes to home-cooked meals from neighbors, and rides home from school for your older kids, or whatever it is that someone offers you. Whether it's in the hospital or in bed with your husband or when your in-laws are over for a visit, just say YES. Hand off that baby if you need a nap, a quick shower, or just a few moments of alone time to take a few deep breaths. These little breaks will become more important as time passes and you get more tired.

"Some women are exhausted right away, depending on what their labor was like," Dr. Bickman said. "That's why I say they should take advantage of the hospital nursery if they need to. Remember, these nurses here are professionals put on earth, or at least on your wing of the hospital, to take care of your baby's every need. You have just gone through a roller coaster of a physical experience and likely missed out on some serious sleep—there's nothing like the uncomfortable last few weeks of pregnancy to rob your body of rest when you need to be stockpiling it most. So if you need a few hours of sleep, take them. And if you want to keep your baby in the room with you while you nod off, even better."

I didn't feel like I needed any help in the hospital, so I kept Titan right at my side 24/7. It was when I got back home that the adrenaline started to wear off and I started to feel just flattened by exhaustion. I would do anything to sneak in an extra hour wherever I could get it, so that time when I passed out on the couch and my friends volunteered to watch Titan for an hour while I grabbed a nap, I took them up on it. How could I not? I knew Titan would survive an hour without me, and I had quickly come to understand that I needed to be firing on all cylinders pretty much around the clock at that point, so the rest I was getting was directly benefiting him, too. It truly does take a village to raise a child. Your friends and loved ones are there to help you, so please—let them!

Sleep Rule 3: Sleep whenever you can.

I also came to embrace the cliché of sleeping when the baby sleeps whenever I could. Newborns do sleep all the time, even if it's not always on the most convenient schedule. So even though you have a million things to do in those hours (wash the huge piles of laundry that such a tiny creature manages to produce, cook food, clean up your nasty kitchen, write thank-you notes for all the wonderful onesies your friends sent, update your address book so you can finally get those birth announcements out, and on and on and on), all of that can wait if you're tired. Just stretch out and stare up at the fan just like your baby loves to do.

I learned pretty early that motherhood is a sprint, not a marathon. The better you take care of yourself today, the better you'll be able to take care of your baby tomorrow, or at two, four, and six in the morning when that demanding little tyrant wants his next meal. So just forget your usual schedule ever existed—you'll get back to it one day. But right now, your baby doesn't know the difference between night and day, so whenever you get a chance to nap, whether it's at ten in the morning or at that time of the day when you're usually walking in from work, take a rest if you need it.

Sleep Rule 4: Don't forget there's a light at the end of the tunnel.

Dr. Bickman put it best: "The fatigue will be unlike anything you've ever experienced, but then before you know it, it'll be over. I can't tell you the number of first-time moms who call me in distress a few days after they've come home with their new baby and say, 'This is so crazy and overwhelming—no one ever told me it was going to be like this! I'm not going to make it!' But in most cases, it's the sleep deprivation talking. I assure them that, no matter how hard it seems at first, they won't always feel this way. And, sure enough, when they come into my office for the six-week postpartum checkup, these women are totally transformed. The baby isn't screaming and waking up so much, they're getting a little more sleep, they've adjusted to nursing, they're no longer in such acute pain. They might even be wearing makeup again! And no matter how impossible it seems right now, your baby will sleep through the night eventually—I swear. No human has ever stayed up all night for eight years."

Dr. Bickman was absolutely right (as usual). Just when I really felt like I was reaching that point of total exhaustion, something amazing happened: Titan started sleeping longer. Unbelievable as it might seem, all babies really do get the hang of the sleep thing at some point. The average is six months, but some start a lot earlier; some not till much later. It depends on how much they weigh and a million other factors. By two and a half months, my guy was sleeping four hours at a stretch, and a few weeks after that, it was six. I'd made it—we'd come out on the other side!

Sleep Rule 5: Never wake a sleeping baby.

The funny thing was that once Titan started sleeping longer, it was like *I'd* lost the habit of sleeping through the night. I was so used to waking up for him at all hours that a few times a night, with no prompting from the crib, I would rocket out of bed with a start. And when I still didn't hear anything, I would creep into his bedroom and check on him, and sometimes I'd sort of give him a tiny push to make sure he would squirm in response.

Dr. Bickman told me that this was a totally normal form of paranoia that grips mothers of infants. "I'm not a pediatrician," she said, "but there's truth in the old cliché to never wake a sleeping baby. That's what my pediatrician told me after my first baby, and I've always followed that advice. If your baby is growing and your doctor isn't worried about his weight gain, let him sleep! Don't wake him every hour, or even every four hours, unless you have a medical reason to do so. Yeah, your baby will probably eat if you offer him your breast every hour, but if someone offered you M&Ms every hour you would probably eat them, too. That doesn't mean you have to, or should. The baby will wake up when he's hungry, and that will probably be sooner than you'd like to wake up, so when he's sleeping, let him. He's not going to starve to death! Nothing bad is going to happen to the baby except that he'll wake up hungry. But something bad will happen to *you* if you insist on getting up every hour all night: you will collapse."

It turns out that this was pretty easy advice to follow! Though it took our bodies a while to readjust to sleeping for longer than an hour and half at a stretch, we eventually got the hang of it again. As soon as I was a little less exhausted, I could barely remember how tired I'd been; it's something you can only experience in the moment. So trust me. No matter how unbelievable it may seem when you have a teeny-tiny around-the-clock-needy newborn, things usually will turn around for you—at least partially—at six to eight weeks. By three months you'll feel even better, and by a year you will (mostly) have adapted to your crazy new life. As with so much else, there is a light at the end of the tunnel. By the time he was six months old, Titan was making it all the way till morning more often than not, and I had fully remembered how much I loved a good night's sleep.

Sleep Rule 6: Relax!

By which I mean, don't just try to cram in sleep at every possible opportunity, but simply *relax* mentally whenever you can. Try to find some inner peace, and cut yourself some slack. Just remember that babies are the most remarkably resilient creatures, and you're not going to ruin your child for life if you feed him ten minutes later than scheduled. This advice applies to so many other things as well. If your baby wears a wet diaper for an extra ten minutes, he will survive it. If he gets a diaper rash, it won't last forever. Just hang on to your perspective, which I understand is much easier said than done when you are crazed with exhaustion, but you can at least make that your goal.

CHAPTER 9

So Now We're Both Wearing Diapers?

(Urinary Incontinence)

I WILL NEVER FORGET sitting down for lunch with a group of friends when Titan was about six weeks old. One of my friends said something that cracked me up, so (naturally) I burst out laughing—and simultaneously peed a little. I thought to myself, "Wow. There goes all my dignity." But Titan was still incredibly tiny, so I decided to give myself a break. I excused myself, darted to the store around the corner, and picked up a new pair of underwear. Done! Nobody would've ever found out about my little indiscretion if I hadn't decided to write about it in this book. That wasn't my only wet-underwear incident, of course. All the time, those first few weeks, when I'd laugh or cough or sneeze or lift a heavy box of diapers or even just get up from the couch too fast, I'd often be rewarded with a thin stream of urine between my legs.

And to think I'd assumed the constant peeing—not a couple of times a day but a couple of times an hour—would end with pregnancy! I mean, there was no longer a gigantic baby literally sitting directly on top of my bladder, so what was going on? Why couldn't I hold my damn pee? I've already written about how heavy I felt when I first got up to use the bathroom after giving birth. Well, I'm here to tell you that that feeling didn't go away for quite some time. Those first weeks, I was literally getting up to go to the bathroom every fifteen minutes. And sometimes when I'd get to the toilet, nothing would come out! I would have to knead on my tummy to release the pee, and even that didn't always work to get things moving down there. Sometimes I felt like I was about to burst and only a tiny trickle would dribble out.

But even though my trips to the toilet could be unpredictable, there was one constant those early weeks: I was always leaking a little in my underwear, often without even knowing it. And while it was most definitely not an enjoyable sensation to realize that the area between my legs was damp with pee again, I eventually accepted that there wasn't really anything I could do about it except stock up on new underwear, and keep that washing machine at work. Seriously, you think the *baby* changes clothes often? Your underwear might also be in constant rotation. But that's okay! That constant leakage is all part of the new-mama package. Still, that didn't stop me from wanting to know what exactly was going on (and when it would stop), so I put a few questions to Dr. Bickman.

Why does it happen?

"It's called stress incontinence," Dr. Bickman said, "and one reason for it is the big fluctuation in hormones you're experiencing. Estrogen strengthens the muscles around the opening of your urethra, particularly the sphincter that holds your urine in. When your estrogen levels drop, your sphincter weakens and that's why you're leaking pee left and right. Estrogen also goes down while you're nursing, which is why the incontinence can sometimes persist for a while. We give patients estrogen cream to put right around the muscles of the urethra to strengthen the muscles there, though it can take a few weeks to work.

"But there's another reason you might have trouble if you've had a vaginal birth, especially if forceps were involved," she said. (Phew—I was spared the forceps this time around!) "All that pushing you had to do to get the baby out has weakened the actual bladder muscle; it's kind of like all the exertion has temporarily sprained it. All the surrounding tissues that are holding your bladder in place have been stretched to their limit, too, so your bladder is still bouncing around in there, which is why sometimes it feels full to bursting even when it's not.

"These pelvic-floor muscles also got a major workout, and they'll require even more recovery time. That means that when you feel a pee coming on and instinctively tighten those muscles to keep it in, they just might not be able to respond like they once did. The other force at work is the shrinking of the uterus, which is positioned directly on top of your bladder. The uterus takes about six weeks to get back to its previous shape, and while it's contracting and shifting, it's disturbing the adjacent pee storage unit, so it's no wonder your bladder is so confused."

But what if you've had a C-section?

My girlfriend never even went into labor and she swears she had the whole trickling-pee thing, too. "That could be from the epidural," Dr. Bickman said. "If you've had a catheter in your bladder, some incontinence can be a common side effect. And when you get a C-section, well, the doctor is physically pushing the bladder away to remove the baby. I am actually touching your bladder with my hands to pull out your little bundle of joy, and that can paralyze the bladder for a time. So it's the same result as when you push for hours, but a slightly different mechanism causing it. It can be a double whammy if you've pushed and then had a C-section anyway, and you might have a longer recovery time."

Anything I can do to return to dry-underwear days faster?

"You could definitely do Kegels if you're so inspired," Dr. Bickman said, referring to the exercises that can strengthen the pelvic-floor muscles. "But you have to do them all the time, or don't bother doing them at all. Unless you're really religious about it, tightening up every time you're at a traffic light, you might as well spare yourself the effort. I'm not saying they don't work—they absolutely do—you just have to be on your game to get any payoff."

To know which muscles Kegels target, try to cut off your pee midflow the next time you're going to the bathroom. Those are the muscles that are causing you to leak pee, and the ones you need to strengthen if you want to put those days behind you. To get them back in shape, you tighten those muscles (and not while you're on the toilet, but when you're in a place where you can concentrate), count to five while holding the contraction, and then release. Relax a few seconds between contractions. Do this up to ten times in a row, holding the contraction a little longer every time until you can hold it for ten consecutive seconds. To see real results, you have to do these rounds of exercises at least three times a day every day. And like Dr. Bickman said, Kegels work, but—speaking from experience here—it is very, very hard to find that quiet time every day to do them.

How long till I get over it?

Dr. B. assured me that within six months my whole peeing situation would be back to normal, and I am happy to report that I can now leave the house without carrying a spare pair of underwear in my diaper bag. The things we measure as progress when we become moms!

"I told you!" Dr. Bickman said. "I know how mortifying it can be when you leak pee right in the middle of your workday, but I've been doing this for seventeen years, and do you know how many times I've had a patient with permanent pee issues? Never. Not even once. Of course it does happen, but it's incredibly rare. Incontinence might revisit you when you're seventy, and that's normal, but it's unlikely to persist between then and now."

CHAPTER 10

Why Can't I Think about Anything but Breastfeeding?

(The Psychological Side of Nursing)

AND NOW TO THE BIG, BIG TOPIC—breastfeeding. You thought I'd forgotten all about it, didn't you? As if that's not the one change that most rocks your world after you give birth, besides the presence of an actual baby outside your body, of course. I know I'm not alone when I confess that, in the days and weeks after giving birth to Titan, I quickly became obsessed—just obsessed—with breastfeeding, even though (or maybe because?) what was supposed to be the most natural act in the world didn't come totally naturally to me. In fact, I found it really, really difficult at first. How had all those cave women managed to keep their babies alive for so many thousands of years? I think I was totally unprepared for just how hard breastfeeding was.

Soon after Titan was born, the pediatrician who examined him in the hospital basically accused me of not feeding my baby enough. "The baby's lost weight," she told me accusingly. "You're obviously not producing enough milk for him." Of course I burst into tears. I was already an emotional wreck after several consecutive days with no sleep, and here this person in a position of authority was making me feel like total shiznit? I was breastfeeding him every hour around the clock and thought it was going fine. What more could I do? Doctors should be careful with words like that—they're shooting loaded guns.

After that scolding from the pediatrician made me feel so inadequate, I started to worry that I was a total failure as a parent. What was wrong with me? Why couldn't I provide for my baby like I needed to? I called a friend who was an experienced mom and she said, "What are you talking about? Just chill—your milk probably hasn't even come in yet!" How was I supposed to know that milk takes three or four days after childbirth to fully show up? That wasn't in any of the books I'd read, and if that was the case, why was that pediatrician so rude about it? And after all, all babies lose weight after they're born. It wasn't like Titan was in any danger of wasting away! I still resent that doctor for making me feel bad about myself when I was at my most vulnerable.

As I learned the hard way while still in the hospital, there is so much judgment out there for women who breastfeed, or can't breastfeed, or give up earlier than intended, and it's just not right. We are all doing the best we can in a huge range of different circumstances, and we all need to go easier on ourselves. If breastfeeding is a cinch, that's great. If it's challenging for you, don't beat yourself up over it. Your ability to breastfeed, or not, is not at all a measure of how well you can mother

For some women, breastfeeding is like breathing. They figure it out instantly, with no preparation or training. But for even more women, there's a hiccup at first, a difficulty to overcome. Most, but by no means all of the time, women get over this hump, but the ones who don't should absolutely not feel bad about themselves. Whenever you need to, give your baby a bottle. The baby will have no memory of it, and the important thing is that you feed your child. Breastfeeding is great, but success at breastfeeding is not a gauge of your success as a mother. If you're having trouble breastfeeding, there are plenty of resources you can use: group classes, free consultants who come to your hospital bed, people who will visit you at home afterward. But if you don't get it down, just remember that it's okay.

I cannot tell you how many patients I've had who have reached insane levels of stress about their difficulties breastfeeding. They call me in tears all the time. Again and again I say the exact same thing: it is not worth it. These people taking Zoloft and going into therapy just because they can't breastfeed? No. Step away. Every time this happens, I just tell my patients to give it up already. You cannot let this one thing ruin your whole experience as a new mom. If it's not working, it's okay. Don't blame yourself! You just delivered your baby; you are a total champ whether you breastfeed or not. Just forget it and go back to staring into your beautiful baby's eyes. You'll probably fail at something else in your life, so just get on with it and focus on your baby and your body's recovery. And no matter what, enjoy your baby. It's such a shame when I see people suffering for their whole maternity leave and then that's it, it's over, they're back at work. They'll never have this time with their newborn again. If they'd just given their babies formula, the babies would've been happy and the mom would've been much less stressed and enjoyed her time with the baby more.

your child. What seems so do-or-die when your child is an infant will not always loom as large in your mind.

Dr. Bickman recommended that I go see a lactation consultant after I got home from the hospital. (Our hospital had a great lactation consultant on staff, but she had so many patients to see that she would only stop by my room for a few minutes at a time.) Even if you think you have it down while you're at the hospital, a lot of times your milk doesn't come in until you're back home, and you may end up feeling totally clueless all over again. "I've given birth five times," Dr. Bickman said, "and I've seen a lactation consultant five times. Sometimes you just need a little bit of hands-on coaching to get you on the right track."

That's how I got hooked up with Linda Hanna, who turned out to be a lifesaving goddess at a time when I really, really needed some nonjudgmental wisdom. Linda is a registered nurse, has a master's in nursing education, and is an international board-certified lactation consultant—basically the whole package from a woman's-health point of view. And she's also a really cool woman. I liked her so much that, even after I got the hang of breastfeeding, I'd keep calling her just to hang out! "Linda," I'd say, "I need you, Titan isn't eating enough!" So she'd come over to check him out and then say, "Look at that big full tummy—he's doing great!" And then I'd be forced to admit that I just wanted to spend some time with her because she made me feel so much calmer and saner. Looking back, I think that part of my attachment to Linda came from the fact that I lost my mom soon after Titan's birth, and she stepped in to provide the maternal wisdom I was so missing in those weeks.

When I told Linda about my plans to write this book, I asked her to give me some of the nursing tips that the women she sees find most helpful. This advice was invaluable for me as I began to navigate the painful, exhausting, but ultimately awesome roller coaster that was breastfeeding.

Tip 1: Know what you want.

"Every situation is very unique and individual, so I wouldn't give everyone the same advice," Linda said. "But every woman needs to have some sense of what it is that she wants to do. Are you exclusively nursing? Are you nursing and pumping and also bottle feeding? Do you want the feeling of nursing but don't really care if the baby only gets your milk? Keep asking: What is it you want? What works for your life? There is no right or wrong answer here—you just have to figure out what's best for you and your family. You can't plan certain things, and you can't plan breastfeeding because you can't have a conversation with a baby either prenatally or after they're born, and you can't always know your own self that well if you've never been on that road before.

"But you *can* try to find your own path, make a concise, easy-to-digest plan that fits into your life, and surround yourself with people who can nurture that. Whether it's a nursing coach or a sister or a friend, you need to find someone you can talk to who understands your story and who can help you in your version of your story and not somebody else's story. It doesn't matter what your neighbor's story or your best friend's story was. You need to focus on a plan that fits in with your life as it is, not as you dreamed it could be.

"Always, always surround yourself with people who are going to help and nurture you and not make you feel bad or like you did something wrong if things don't go exactly as you imagined—and this doesn't just apply to breastfeeding. Bring your core team together, share with them what you want, what they could help you do, and then accept their help. If you start from there, you will be much more accepting of what your journey is going to look like even if it turns out nothing like you planned."

(Do you see why I love this woman?)

Tip 2: Today is one day only, and one day isn't forever.

"Try not to get too wrapped up in the symbolism of today, because no matter what happens, tomorrow is another day and maybe then we'll make more milk, or maybe then we'll decide to wean. Just deal with the present moment, because every day we can tweak things and revisit them and take another look. Maybe you're tired one morning and not so tired the next morning, and that gives you a different outlook. Don't let yourself feel stuck. Look forward but always with a positive attitude, knowing that what happened yesterday is in the past; it's done. If something you tried didn't work, it doesn't matter. You can always try something new tomorrow.

"If you had a whole list of things you wanted to accomplish today—maybe you missed a pumping session, or you didn't do skin-to-skin for as long as you intended—and you suddenly discover that it's already almost dinnertime and you didn't accomplish most of the list, it's okay. Just tell yourself that tomorrow is another chance to start fresh. You didn't miss anything; you didn't fail at any essential task. If it didn't get done today, then it didn't need to get done."

I had to remind myself of this one all the time because I never produced as much milk as I thought Titan needed, and it was hard not to get frustrated and decide to give up when I'd tried every single trick in the book and still just got a little bit of milk. But though my instinct was to feel bad and beat myself up about it, Linda helped steer me away from that type of negative, self-defeating thinking.

Tip 3: Take care of yourself.

"Maintaining your own health and sanity—getting enough rest, and food, and downtime—is absolutely crucial to this process," Linda told me. "However busy you are, however much you have on your plate—and this generation of mothers takes on a lot—you need to take a moment of meditation and remind yourself that you can't do everything all the time. Having a baby is hard, but it's particularly hard when you're a high achiever who's used to doing everything exactly right all the time. Because that baby comes in and just turns everything upside down and you can no longer accomplish every single thing on your checklist. But that's okay."

This one, for me, was hard at first. I am a bit of a perfectionist, and I love running the show. But after Titan was born, I began to realize that I just couldn't have my hand in every pie, at least not for a little while. If I wanted to get the hang of this new-mom thing—and part of that was breastfeeding, but not all of it—I had to really relinquish control for a while and let Tim and my visiting friends and my amazing assistant take the steering wheel, whether it was about figuring out what we were doing for dinner or making sure the laundry got done or calling our insurance company about the hospital stay. Though it went against my essential Type A nature, I just had to surrender control of all the details and focus on the baby.

Tip 4: Rely on your support network.

"I'm always telling new moms to know that they have support around them and to call for help whenever they need it," Linda said. "You may not know every single thing just yet, but you do know more than you think, and you know your baby better than anybody. But if something doesn't feel right, ask for help. Letting people help you is a huge part of the story.

"Breastfeeding itself isn't really hard," Linda kept reminding me. "It's all the other little things you have to do while you're nursing the baby that can feel so daunting. Preparing meals. Getting rest. Having an opportunity to pump. Getting out to the grocery store. Again, that's why you have to ask the people around you who want to be with you on the journey as long as you need them, knowing that they've been included and are valuable. Then you can just ask, 'Hey, can you pick up some milk for me on your way home?' and know it won't be an issue. Just one less thing on your list."

Tip 5: Remember that you're a winner no matter what.

"Every once in a while, recheck your goals. What did you want out of this experience? What does your baby need? What were your original goals? If they haven't panned out exactly as you imagined it, recheck yourself. Work with what you can and what you have, and love this special relationship that you get to have with your baby, whether you're breastfeeding or breast-milk-feeding or formula-feeding. There are so many legitimate ways to feed the baby, and once you've found one that works for you—and that way may be completely different from what works for the woman next door or even what worked for you with your previous baby—then you're a winner. We're living in this life and we're going to do the best we can with what we have, so don't put unnecessary pressure on yourself in this vulnerable time."

Linda was so amazing because she was all about nurturing the mother, being kind and loving to her. "We have to be friendly to mothers first. We're not nice to them. We judge them, we criticize them, we make them do things that they don't feel ready to do, and we have to start being kinder and gentler and nicer to someone who's just gone through an entire year of her life changed forever. Mothers need to know that anything they do is a win in the world of babies. Every single day is a win. Maybe not every day went exactly as you thought it should go, but it's a win for you and your husband and your baby and everyone who is on that journey with you. So stop looking for things that aren't there and love and embrace the things that are there." Amen to that!

Once I had Linda in my life, I felt like I could really move forward with my breastfeeding goals. The one-day-at-a-time mantra really helped me, especially in those first few weeks when I literally got *no* sleep because Titan was hungry all the time. I was so excited to be a new mother and so excited to provide milk for my baby that I didn't really take into account how often Titan would eat. By the third week I was like, "Can we pump now?" In the end, that's what I started doing in the evenings so I could sleep through one of the many, many night feedings, and I'm so glad I was able to make that choice. I was feeding my baby the best I could, and that made me a winner.

Even so, those early weeks, as I got more psychologically adjusted to the demands of breastfeeding, I wasn't prepared for how taxing it would be on my body.

CHAPTER 11

Are My Boobs Always Going to Be Like This?

(The Physical Side of Breastfeeding)

Now, NO DISCUSSION of breastfeeding would be complete without getting into the nitty-gritty realities of what it does to your body. In a nutshell: your boobs change shape, your nipples turn into UFOs, your hunger is insatiable—the list goes on and on.

But the first and most important thing is that breastfeeding can hurt. A LOT. When I complained to Dr. Bickman about the pain in my nipples that first week—how could a tiny baby cause so much pain when he didn't even have teeth yet?—she told me that it was nature's way of distracting me from the pain in my vagina. Fair enough.

A lot of moms experience serious discomfort while still figuring out the whole latch situation—and it takes a while for your boobs to get used to it!—but it will gradually subside, or at least it's supposed to. Like so many aspects of postpartum life, pain is part of the package, but it should decrease, not increase with every passing day. Linda gave me something called APNO cream (all-purpose nipple ointment), just in case my nipples started to hurt. She told me I should get back to her if I experienced any of the following symptoms (which, luckily, I did not):

- Irritation gets worse, not better.
- Your boobs start to change color.
- You get a fever.
- The standard pain medicine you were taking stops working all of a sudden.

I remember when I got breast implants, I felt really nervous that I wouldn't be able to breastfeed later on, but when my time came, I could still get my two ounces out when I needed to, and I have friends with implants who got an abundance of milk.

So while in some ways I was pleasantly surprised by my ability to produce milk, I still had trouble adjusting to some of the physical changes that accompanied breastfeeding. These were the main ones.

Get ready for some major hunger.

Yeah, yeah, I know, you want to drop those fifty pounds and be red-carpet ready overnight but, girl—just relax. If you're breastfeeding, you are going to be starving all the time. I just could not eat often enough, which I guess makes sense when you consider that the baby you're feeding is gaining weight so rapidly after he's out in the world, and if you're exclusively breastfeeding he's relying on you for all his nutrition, only now he weighs ten pounds instead of six. So get ready, because pregnancy hunger's got nothing on breastfeeding hunger.

RECOMMENDED HERBS

There are herbs you can take to increase lactation success. I religiously took the ones Linda recommended, those first several months. They fall into two main categories.

The ones that actually make more milk. These herbs are known as galactagogues, because they produce more breast milk by stimulating the alveoli to secrete more. Popular galactagogues include goat's rue, moringa, and malunggay. But while these herbs can be great at increasing production, they can also make your dopamine, the so-called happy hormone, levels go down a bit and can leave you feeling depressed, so don't take these without the advice of a professional, especially if you have a history of depression.

The ones that help squeeze out the milk that's already there. These include fenugreek, shatakari, blessed thistle, and nettle. This category of herbs enhances levels of the hormone oxytocin, which squeezes the alveoli where the milk is stored, and that process helps push more milk out of every gland. So while it looks like you're getting more milk, you're really just doing a better job of extracting the milk you already have.

I tried to eat foods that would promote milk production without irritating the baby's tummy. I ate my oatmeal every morning and snacked on lactation cookies and was just really careful about what I put in my body because I didn't want the baby to have gas. I didn't eat raw food or any of the stuff they tell you to stay away from. I pretty much stuck to the menu Linda gave me, which meant minimal dairy, spicy foods, corn, eggs, and soy. I found that you could kind of mix it up and see what worked and what didn't those first few weeks. And because I was so invested in upping my milk production, I tried to build my diet around the foods that Linda said would help me get out more milk:

- Alfalfa
- Barley
- Wheatgrass
- Quinoa
- Coconut

Linda also recommended bone broth, which apparently improves the quality of breastmilk, making it richer and creamier, but I never got to try that!

MAKE YOUR OWN BONE BROTH

Making bone broth (which is very hard to find in stores) sounded intimidating to me, but once Linda explained how easy it is, I wish I'd tried to whip some up. I will definitely make it for my next child! Basically, all you do is go to the butcher counter of your grocery store and ask them for some leftover bones; they will usually just give them to you, or charge you very little. Then you put the bones on the stove and boil them for at least six hours—the same thing you'd do to make broth with your Thanksgiving turkey leftovers—and continually remove liquid that has been infused with the bones. Along the way, you can add any seasonings you'd like as well as vegetables, chicken, or other meat to flavor the broth to your liking. Just experiment as you go, and have fun with it!

You will also be really, really, really thirsty.

You need to have buckets of water around you at all times those early weeks, both for the bloating situation we've already discussed, and because your throat will feel like the Sahara Desert and you will not be able to drink enough water. Even if you've never been an avid water drinker in your life to date, do yourself, and your baby, a favor by getting in the habit of chugging water around the clock.

You will leak at the most unexpected times.

If you thought you'd just be leaking blood and pee those first weeks, think again: your boobs want in on the action too. Get ready for your breasts to be leaking everywhere, around the clock. A good nursing bra will help this situation. Linda recommended that I get a nice variety for different uses, so I tried a mix of bras from Elle MacPherson, Medela, and Bravado; some I wore for work, some I wore at home, and some I even slept in. I just mixed it up until I found what worked. But even with the perfect nursing bra and nice, thick nursing pads, you can expect some big symmetrical circles on your shirt if you're not emptying those boobs every couple of hours (and in fact even if you are). You will be amazed at all the dripping they'll do!

You need a comfortable spot where you can relax.

Get a nice comfy chair, some breastfeeding pillows, maybe with a table right next to you where you can load up on magazines—and don't forget to have a bottle of water handy. Keep your remote control and iPad handy, too! If you're going to be pumping, you need some of those hands-free bras so that you don't have to hold the plastic pump parts right up against your boobs.

Your boobs aren't going to be all that pretty for a while.

Well, actually, they will get nice and full and look like inflatable porn-star boobs for a while (which is why you'll be wearing nursing bras around the clock), but get ready, for their appearance will soon take a major turn for the worse. All that gnawing at your nipples will take its toll! In those early days, I was fascinated (my polite way of saying "horrified") by the transformation of my boobs. My nipples were HUGE—we are talking the size of Frisbees—and sometimes I could see these veins bulging out while I was nursing. My boobs themselves were so long and stretchy that I sometimes felt like I could've slung them over my shoulders. In my pre-mama life, I'd always been really proud of my boobs (well, at least after I got some silicone put in them), but they were no longer the perfect girls

CAN I GET PREGNANT AGAIN WHILE BREASTFEEDING?

The short answer is yes, so I recommend that patients get back on birth control once they've started having sex again. You're always going to have that one ovulation that precedes your first period, and you have no idea when that could happen. Even if you've had a baby before and never got your period while breastfeeding, you could still get one this time around. I've gone from not having a period until three months after breastfeeding to getting one right in the middle of breastfeeding. Every pregnancy is totally different, which is why you need birth control at six weeks, unless of course you're ready to welcome another baby within the year.

they used to be—far from it. Even with the silicone action, it was like some of the air had been sucked out and they just sort of hung there like flapjacks. But, hey, I tried to tell myself, if my perky little girls didn't quite have the same bounce they used to, then I could deal. After all, that's why God created push-up bras. And I can't speak for everyone, but I know I'm going to see someone (wink, wink) after I have my second kid. In the meantime, I just tried to enjoy my ability to feed my baby!

Your boobs probably aren't going to feel very sexual, either.

Another change I noticed was that my boobs just didn't feel sexual anymore. Even after we started having sex again (and that took a while!), I didn't want Tim anywhere near my boobs;

it was as if they existed exclusively to feed my baby, not to excite my husband (as if these big floppy pancakes I was lugging around were all that exciting to anyone). Dr. Bickman warned me that that feeling could last until I was done breastfeeding, which turned out to be the case for me.

In the end, for all the bumps along the way, I completely loved breastfeeding Titan. But when I was done, yes, I admit it: I did a little dance. I'd met my goal and now I could move on to the next amazing phase of parenting!

CHAPTER 12

What Is This Thing Hanging Off My Stomach?

(The Post-Pregnancy Bod)

You know those women who have a baby and stroll out of the hospital the next day in their size 2 jeans? Well, I was not one of them. And while my brain understood that very few women fall into that category (no matter what we see in *Us Weekly*), my heart still had a lot of trouble accepting my new body after the baby had left it.

I mean, when you're pregnant, it makes sense. You're carrying a whole baby in there—of course your body is going to be bigger! But afterward, when the baby is out in the world? I guess part of me expected my body to snap back instantaneously, though in retrospect that's clearly ridiculous. Still, at the time, I would feel a little start of surprise every time I looked in the mirror. I swear I hardly recognized the tired, puffy woman staring back at me.

Of course I understood that it was all normal, that you don't miraculously get your old body back the same day you give birth, but that doesn't mean I was prepared for some of the bigger changes, particularly my stretched-out stomach and boomerang boobs. Just as I tried not to think about how I'd once posed on the cover of *Shape,* I tried not to look too hard at the stretch marks covering my belly. But still I couldn't stop myself from wondering, over and over, "How the hell am I going to get rid of these?" My stomach was loose and floppy and appeared totally detached from my body. Even my feet looked puffy and misshapen. Nothing was how it used to be.

For the first couple of months, my self-esteem was really in the pits about my body. I'd study myself in the mirror and remember what my face looked like when I was smaller, and I'd just feel depressed. I couldn't help it! And then, whenever I weighed myself, the misery deepened. Hadn't I just pushed out a seven-and-a-half-pound baby? And what about all the blood and other nasty stuff that was pouring out of me 24/7? I thought for sure I would've lost half the weight within the first week, but nope.

When I was feeling really down, I reminded myself of how incredibly lucky I was to be in this position at all. There are thousands of women out there who struggle with infertility, and I had gotten pregnant right away and carried a perfect baby to term. I shouldn't be sweating the small stuff! It had taken my body nine months to grow that wonderful baby I was now holding; I really shouldn't expect all evidence of that transformation to vanish overnight.

Don't worry about those women whose bodies miraculously return to their previous bikini-ready condition a day after childbirth—their vaginas probably look *much* worse than yours! But really, nobody emerges from childbirth looking exactly the same as before. We all recover and we all lose weight on our time lines, so it's best to just let our bodies do their thing in the weeks right after birth. In all likelihood, you will end up looking very similar to what you looked like before you got pregnant, but for most people it takes some time. The older you are, the more time it's likely to take.

So what I said about your vagina is the same thing I'll say about the scale: just stay away for the first weeks after birth. Who cares what you weigh at six weeks? I almost always advise my patients, unless they have some condition or I suspect there might be a problem, not to worry about their weight just yet. Unbelievable as it may seem right now, you *will* lose the weight. Trust me, I know how disheartening it is to push out an eight-pound baby and step on the scale to find you've only lost five pounds. But there's nothing you can do about it immediately after birth, so try not to obsess. Just look at Kelly now! There is no way that she was going to be thirty pounds overweight for long; that's not who she is. So it's better not to put that unnecessary pressure on yourself in a time when you're not even allowed to exercise. We always say nine months on, nine months off, but I never thought that was fair. I really think it's more like a year to get your old body back. So give yourself that full year, and if you're still overweight at that point, then you can talk to your doctor about making some changes.

Right. Had to keep my priorities straight and remember what was really important. So while going on a diet seemed tempting, at least in theory, I was more focused on filling up my body with good nutrients to nourish Titan. (And, P.S., it's *really* hard to restrict your caloric intake when you're averaging two hours a night of sleep.) As I've already mentioned, I was starving the whole time I was breastfeeding, so it wasn't like I could've restricted calories even if I'd tried.

"Everyone wants to go on a diet the minute the baby comes out," Dr. Bickman said. "But you really shouldn't because now you're feeding an even bigger baby, and that baby is really relying on the nutrients in what you're eating. So as long as you keep breastfeeding, you're going to burn a lot more calories, and the weight will come off."

I kept repeating that advice to myself, and I tried not to be too daunted by what seemed like a long, impossible journey back to my old body.

Focus on something you love about your new body.

Here's the thing. When you're pregnant, everyone is always cooing over you, telling you how glowing and beautiful you look, and making you feel special even if you're just waiting in line at the grocery store. You get used to being the center of attention whenever you walk into a room. But when the pregnancy is over? Forget about it. You're no longer carrying the baby, and you're just trapped in this body that you've never seen before.

Women get really, really freaked out about the so-called mother's apron, that extra flabby skin that hangs off the stomach post-baby. I had a patient come to me the other day and say, "Look at me, my baby is ten months and I still have all this skin here, it must be a tumor!" Without trying to be mean, I told her that it was just her skin, but she didn't buy it. "What do you mean? It's so firm, it has to be something scary!" She thought it was her uterus or her muscles separating. I said, "No, your muscles are actually tight, you're just carrying extra weight still, which is fine, but don't go confusing a little extra fat with a tumor."

To boost my spirits, I tried to focus on something I loved about my new body—say, my newly rounded booty and my, um, voluptuous hips. I also just tried to be a lot more loving and forgiving of myself, so I would repeat things to myself like, "It's okay. I'm going to live in this beautiful body and build it back up for a year. I sacrificed it and carried this child for nine months and now I'm going to take my time and recover. I'm going to work out and eat healthy, so I can be the best mom and the best person that I can be."

Embrace your new reality—and your new body.

Yes, I was a little thicker than I was before, and nobody was going to ask me to pose on the cover of *Shape* in my first year post-baby, but I also had this precious tiny human to show for the extra couple of inches around my waist. If that was the necessary trade-off, then I was more than happy to spend a few more months in yoga pants. It wasn't like I was going to any fancy dinners with a newborn, anyway. I tried to think of my new body as this amazing proof of everything I'd accomplished as a mom and woman, battle scars and all.

Don't obsess.

There is so much else to drive you crazy in those first few months of motherhood. Is my baby sleeping enough? Or maybe too much? Is his latch correct? Is he too gassy? Oh, no, what do I do if he rolls onto his stomach while he's asleep? Let's let this one little preoccupation drop for the time being. It's not like you're allowed to exercise those first few weeks anyway, so just try to embrace your floppy boobs and luscious fat rolls (I know, I know, easier said than done) and spend your rare free moments gazing into your baby's beautiful eyes rather than scrutinizing those stretch marks.

I learned to roll with these changes the crazy first few months after Titan was born, but when he got older, I was surprised that I still didn't look more like myself again. For the life of me I could not get rid of my stretch marks, and when Titan was almost a year old and a fan posted that photo on Instagram, of me on the cover of *Shape,* I couldn't help but cry a little about my former body, which at the time was in some graveyard somewhere. Before baby, I'd always loved wearing cute little midriffs, but no matter how hard I tried, my stomach still just didn't look the same. My breasts looked a little deflated, like someone had let the air out of them. But I couldn't do anything about that except keep trying to eat right and showing up at the gym day after day. Obsessing over everything that had changed wasn't productive, so I tried to put a lid on it.

Get a new (temporary) wardrobe.

Yes, I know it sounds superficial, but it can be depressing to open your closet and realize that you don't have a single thing that you can throw on in the morning. And obviously the absolute last thing you want to do after having a baby is put on your maternity clothes ever again—or at least not until the next baby is in the oven. There's always an in-between period when your regular clothes are too tight but you'd rather set fire to that maxi dress you wore every day for your third trimester than put it on again.

I talked to my friend, celebrity stylist Rebecca Gross, about what to wear while you're impatiently waiting for your old body to magically reappear. Following Rebecca's simple advice made a huge difference in how I felt about my body during my first year of motherhood.

Step 1: Get Some Jeans

"After about two months, when you're starting to emerge from that newborn zone of never really leaving the house and wearing the same black leggings and T-shirt every single day, you start to feel ready to return to your old self, but unfortunately your body might not be so ready. In those months when you can't fit into your old clothes yet but are done with the leggings, you need to shop for a few items of clothing that fit the current version of your body. Your first order of business is to get some jeans that fit you so you can feel dressed when you leave the house.

"Leggings have their purposes, but at a certain point you want to be in normal clothes again, and jeans are a great place to start. Nice jeans that fit your new body are both versatile—you can dress them up or down—and fashionable. High-waisted jeans are particularly flattering because they really hold your tummy in. You won't feel like you're spilling out of them, or that you're exposing a part of your body that still makes you self-conscious. Just make sure you get a pair that fits."

Step 2: Accentuate the Positive

"Instead of worrying about those ripples in your stomach, accentuate other parts of your body that might be even sexier post-baby. So go ahead and rock your new cleavage. Wear a plunge blouse that doesn't emphasize your waist or your middle section, but draws attention to your new and improved boobs. Then just throw a sleek blazer or jacket over it and you're ready for a night out; no one will be thinking about what your stomach looks like, I promise."

Step 3: Wear Clothes That Fit

"I really cannot emphasize this enough. So many women try to squeeze into their old clothes too soon after baby, and even when they technically fit, they're often unflattering because they're pinching in the wrong places. So don't try to squeeze into a 4 or a 6 because you used to be a 4 or a 6. If after baby you're a 10, get a 10, because wearing the right size will look a lot better than forcing your body into an article of clothing that's too small for you.

"Embracing your in-between size doesn't mean you won't eventually lose the weight. So much of our preoccupation with how we look post-baby is mental and emotional. You don't feel like yourself anymore, and you're afraid you'll never feel sexy, or comfortable, or confident again. The media is always shoveling these unrealistic ideals down our throats with pictures of women who are 'snapping back' and showing off a perfect six-pack a week after giving birth. We need more pictures of what normal women look like, and more realistic expectations of how long it really takes to lose the weight. Women who think, 'In four months, I want to be back to my pre-baby weight' are setting themselves up for disappointment—unless they got that lucky DNA. Give yourself a year in your high-waisted jeans and low-cut blouses, and try to love the body you're in."

Remember, everyone's body is different!

I felt so much better after I picked out a few basic items that would tide me over until I could squeeze back into my old clothes. It helped me accept that "This is what my reality is right now, and that's okay."

CHAPTER 13

Can I Airbrush My Actual Body?
(Skin and Hair Changes)

OH, MAN, and I thought the shape of my body was a trip? I haven't even gotten into the surface of it. We are talking acne, darkened nipples, stretch marks galore, clumps of hair clogging the shower drain every morning, and all sorts of other not at all attractive transformations that I did not see coming. My skin was stretched out all over my abdomen, and the skin of my face was all dry and flakey. When I complained to my dermatologist about this last condition, she simply shrugged and said, "What can I tell you? The absolute worse thing a woman can do to her skin is have a baby." Needless to say, I stopped seeing that dermatologist immediately!

I do want to run through the various changes that your skin and hair undergo after pregnancy. Like many of these changes, some go back to normal fairly soon; others you just have to see as the price of having given birth to such a precious little baby.

Surface Change: Spider Veins

We've already talked about the big bulging varicose veins on the butt, also known as hemorrhoids, that can plague women during and after pregnancy. Spider veins, so called because they look like a little blue web right beneath your skin, are more of a normal part of aging that pregnancy can aggravate. "Spider veins are really superficial, the result of leaking valves," Dr. B. said. "And I'm afraid to say, but they usually don't go away spontaneously. You could try asking your dermatologist about compression hose or, if you're more hard core, injections. Or you could just try to accept that once you've got them, you've got them."

Surface Change: Stretch Marks

When I was pregnant, I slapped cocoa butter all over my body 24/7 because somehow I thought that would help keep my skin supple and prevent stretch marks. I was walking around like a greasy chicken, but no one told me until the very end that I should be taking vitamin C to help build skin elasticity. So of course when I looked down at my stomach after Titan came out, I couldn't help but think that I should've taken more vitamin C, or moisturized even more aggressively.

Dr. B. said that she tells patients to use this Mustela cream called Stretch Marks Double Action. "It worked for me, but again, it's hard to say if it's the product or just genetics. But sometimes people feel better being told that a product will help them, so that's the one I recommend." My amazing facialist, Shani Darden, said she usually recommends that women worried about stretch marks get a Retinol prescription from their dermatologist. "That will really help lighten them a lot," she said. But not enough for me!

I admit it, my stretch marks drove me absolutely crazy. They still do, in fact. Everyone told me they'd go away, but it's just not true! Even though I am (finally) back to my pre-pregnancy size, I still have these stripes all over my stomach and I don't know if I'll ever be able get rid of them. I went to a fancy dermatologist in Beverly Hills and he promised he could get rid of them with this high-tech laser treatment, but three expensive treatments later and I've yet to see real progress.

While the stretch marks are definitely lighter, they are undeniably still there on my belly, and I'm still not sure how much is the lasers and how much is just time. I'm beginning to accept that all the fancy technology in the world just pales in comparison to DNA. Dr. B. agreed: "Stretch marks are probably more genetic than what you do or don't rub on your skin. There are plenty of people out there who use zero products and get no stretch marks at all—we hate those people! But remember, they have really ugly vaginas, so you can't have it all."

Oh, well. I'd just carried around a baby inside my body for almost a year; the stretch marks are a badge of honor that remind me of how motherhood has transformed my body. (Yeah, yeah, yeah—I know, I have trouble falling for that, too!)

Surface Change: Dryness

My whole life, I've taken pride in my clear skin, which I inherited from my grandmother. But after I had Titan, I couldn't believe what happened to the surface of it. My complexion was just really flat and dry, completely without shine or life, and I could see every single nick and scar I'd ever had. When I was pregnant, I moisturized my face as religiously as I did the rest of my body, switching to all-natural products with ingredient names I could pronounce. I was wary of using anything that might hurt my baby, so along with cocoa butter, I used jojoba oil and tons and tons of coconut oil. Coconut oil was my absolute best friend; you could've thrown me in a fryer and I would've turned into a chicken—I was just that soaked in it from head to toe. I used it on my skin and in my hair, everywhere.

But afterward, with my skin so flat and flavorless, I went through a bunch of different products in the hope of bringing my grandmother's dope skin back. In the end, I found that my skin sort of recovered on its own—but it certainly took long enough. In the meantime, I asked Shani for product recommendations, and she told me to hold off on any harsh products until I was done breastfeeding, since they weren't likely to do much to help me.

"Eczema is really common in the aftermath of childbirth," she said, "but like so many of the changes, you just sort of have to wait it out and let your skin recover on its own." It was a combination of getting back into a regular sleep schedule and having my hormones go back to normal that finally restored my complexion. And, yes, I admit that once Titan was off the boob, I went back (shoulder shrug) to my regimen of unpronounceable ingredients.

Surface Change: Nipples

Yep, it's not enough that your nipples have gotten all huge and swollen from the physical pressure of the baby's mouth stretching them to the limit (and I'm sorry to say, but you might be stuck with these mega-nipples for the long haul), but your nipples have changed colors, too. Mine got a lot darker, and when I asked Dr. B. what was up, she told me that it was the usual culprit responsible for so many of the changes your body undergoes during pregnancy and afterward: hormones, hormones, and more hormones.

"After birth, these hormones can trigger an increase in the production of melanin, the pigment that gives your skin, hair, and eyes their color," Dr. Bickman said. "Parts of your body that might already contain higher concentrations of melanin, like your freckles and, yes, your nipples, might suddenly get darker. Other areas, like the ridge above your lip or your cheekbones, can darken abruptly as well, particularly if you're darker skinned to begin with. Sometimes your skin and nipples return to their previous color; sometimes they don't. You might also get little skin tags on your nipples, but these growths of skin are benign, yet another byproduct of your out-of-whack estrogen levels.

"And speaking of hormones, your nipples can also start sprouting random pieces of hair. In most cases, these will disappear once your hormones have gotten back to normal, but if not, just get out your tweezers and keep calm!"

Surface Change: Acne

Remember that sexy glow your skin had during pregnancy? Well, now it's gone, replaced with some seriously nasty acne. That's right—acne! Your teenage body is gone forever, but not, it seems, your teenage complexion. Dr. Bickman explained to me that the acne that shows up after baby comes from the plunge in estrogen after you give birth. Shani also told me that she sees it a lot, and that some of her clients come in for more facials than usual in those up-and-down weeks. But, unfortunately, there's not much you can do about it except wait it out. Drinking lots of water to flush out your skin also helps, yet another reason to keep chugging down water all day even if it means (sigh) that you have pee constantly trickling down your leg. It's better than huge pimples all over your face!

In terms of products, there's again no amazing quick-fix miracle worker that you can apply; because the cause of the acne is hormonal, no topical product will make that much of a difference. As with so much else, you just have to ride it out and deal with the breakouts until your hormone levels have stabilized.

Surface Change: Melasma

Melasma is the term for those random spots of brown that randomly crop up all over your skin. You know what I'm talking about. Your skin darkens around your lip, right at your mustache line, or you have a little rash around your eyes that makes it look as if you've been in a boxing match. So, yeah, in addition to all your other problems, you might look like you've grown a mustache and been punched in the eye—very attractive, I know. But the good news, according to Dr. B., is that this melasma is both very common and in most cases very temporary.

She told me, "When you're expecting, you get an estrogen overload, which produces that famous pregnancy glow, but you're also producing more melanin, the hormone that pigments skin, and that can lead to some dark splotches on your face that can become more noticeable after the baby comes out. That's because as your skin is contracting and the puffiness is receding, the discoloration suddenly becomes much more obvious, which of course makes women totally self-conscious."

But fear not! Dr. B. assured me that the melasma eventually fades, "though it may not be until after you're done breast-feeding. In the meantime, you should keep your skin protected from the sun, and remember that the spots might come back, just like fat." She said bleaching creams should wait until after breastfeeding, and reminded me that, like so many of the horrific-seeming things that happen to our bodies post-baby, melasma is a pretty small problem to have in the grand scheme of things. "If that's the worst thing that happens to you, you're fine. You can deal with it later."

Shani agreed. She said that a ton of her clients call her about the brown spots that appear on their skin, and that every time she just has to tell them that they can't do anything about it until they're done breastfeeding. "It's pointless to get laser while your hormones are still in flux like that," she said. "You have to give your skin a chance to see if it's going to go back on its own."

Surface Change: Linea Nigra

The linea nigra is the line of fine dark hair that goes from the bottom of your belly button down to your lady parts. This hair, yet another byproduct of all the estrogen and other hormones flooding your system while you're pregnant, tends to get thicker and darker as your pregnancy progresses. It's as if its length mimics the number of weeks of your pregnancy. As it grows, so does the uterus, until it's practically reached the bottom of your sternum.

What was up with this random hair growth? "Remember how your body starts pumping out more melanin than usual when you're pregnant and your skin gets darker in these random patches?" Dr. Bickman said when I posed the question to her. "The same process is at work with the linea nigra. By the end, it might be so thick and dark that an astronaut could see it from space. It will probably go back to normal within a few months after giving birth, but if not, there's always bleach."

Surface Change: Loose Skin

Oh, yeah, you know what I'm talking about! Just as you start to lose weight and feel good about your bod again, your skin gets all loose and floppy, like a sheet attached to your body. Again, this is totally normal. Sometimes, when your body gets bigger and then smaller again, there's extra skin left over. This is particularly true if you've had twins or triplets; your body has been stretched to the limit, and so has your skin. Exercise can be great at firming skin back up and helping it recover, but it can't do everything; I have two girlfriends with insane six-pack abs, and they've *still* got that extra skin. You can also eat extra protein to help build up your collagen levels and firm your skin up, but again—you still might not be able to obliterate those extra flaps. So just do all you can do in terms of exercise (which we'll talk about) and nutrition and hope for the best, but don't expect miracles. Sometimes the extra skin is here to stay, and I promise you that's okay. If it's really bad, get a one-piece! Most of the time, though, your abs will go pretty much back to normal.

Surface Change: Hair Loss

This is one of the most widely publicized, but probably one of the least big-deal, changes that scare new moms. At about three months postpartum, you might notice that you're shedding lots and lots of hair. Your hairbrush is suddenly filled with hair, and you notice clumps of hair clogging your shower drain.

Here's why it's happening. At any given time, you are shedding between 5 and 15 percent of your hair; you may lose about a hundred hairs every day without even noticing. When you're pregnant and your estrogen levels spike, the normal hundred-hair-a-day loss goes on hiatus, and suddenly your hair looks super lush and amazing. Think of it as nature giving you an extra-dope hairdo to compensate for what's going on in other recently expanded regions of your bod.

But don't get too used to your luxuriant new tresses, because when baby arrives and your estrogen levels plummet, your thick hair starts falling out in big scary bunches. But however dramatic the hair loss seems, you will not end up with less hair than you had pre-pregnancy. You are just returning to your usual hair quantities. I know, I know—I loved my thick hair too! But I promise that you don't have to start looking into female toupees, because you should have your regular amount of hair back by the time baby blows out his first birthday candle.

I asked Dr. Bickman if there was anything I could do to stop the shedding, and she said no. "You really just have to wait it out, but if you've been thinking about going for a dramatic new pixie do, now might be a good opportunity. Dye it, pull it back into a ponytail, whatever—I suggest something low maintenance in a time when you're already so busy with the new baby."

She also said that some women's hair sticks around for a while longer before falling out. "In some cases, you may keep your extra hair until you're done breastfeeding, so it might come as even more of a surprise when the hair starts falling off a long time after the newborn phase. Whenever it happens, it's the same hormonal process at work: estrogen takes a nosedive, and hairs follow. The hair loss has nothing to do with any nutritional deficiencies, but of course you should still be taking your prenatal vitamin while your whole body is getting back on track."

CHAPTER 14

Why Can't I Sit Down without Wincing?

(Aches and Pains)

You THINK the head-to-toe pain ends with the pushing? I did, too—and I had some big surprises in store for me. Most women get aches and pains in all sorts of strange places for weeks or even months after childbirth.

Before Titan was born, I had this unbelievably intense pain that spread across my entire pelvic region. I couldn't even walk around toward the end because it hurt so bad. My doula came over and helped me breathe through it, and my physical therapist had me do random breathing techniques and certain stretches, but the pain persisted as long as the baby was inside me.

Afterward, this pain, which seemed so all consuming, got better on its own, allowing me to direct all my attention to the pain in my torn-up vagina. But I wasn't out of the woods yet. When Titan was just under a year old, I developed a persistent pain in my tailbone and started getting massages to treat it. One look at my coccyx and my massage therapist said, "You did this when you gave birth." In subsequent months, I've been going to physical therapy, but even now, I still can't sit in uncushioned chairs for more than a few minutes without having to reposition myself.

Then, when Titan was about one and a half, I started to get some twinges in my neck that I'm sorry to say I totally ignored. I remember somebody once telling me, "When you're feeling achy, your body is telling you that something is up." But I just tried to forget about the pain until a few days later, when I was getting ready for the BET Awards. I had my hair and makeup all done and I was walking over to put on my dress when all of a sudden I felt the most excruciating pain—we are talking worse than labor pains. I tried over and over to put my dress on, but I couldn't move my back. Lucky for me, a good friend of mine, Juliet Barnes, who's a certified athletic trainer and health-care professional who works with athletes at Northwestern University, happened to be in town for the summer. The afternoon of the BET Awards, she came over and found me in tears. "You're not going anywhere," she said and literally picked me up and took me to bed. "You can't move, and how do you expect to stand up in heels?" Then I remembered the day before, when I'd worn heels the whole day despite the pain in my back.

I was completely immobilized for more than a day; I just absolutely could not move. My beautiful, gorgeous dress a designer had made just for me remained on the hanger. When Juliet came over the next day and found me still in bed, I told her that I couldn't figure out what was wrong with me. I'd had an MRI, but the doctors hadn't found anything; my spine had looked perfectly aligned. So then Juliet performed a test on me. I turned over and she asked me to breathe and then flex the muscles of my core. When I did that, to my horror, she stuck three fingers in between my abs and said, "This has been your problem all along!"

It turned out that I had diastasis recti, which refers to the separation of the two main abdominal muscles right down the middle of my core. It's apparently a fairly common problem that can affect as many as two-thirds of pregnant women, but I hadn't even *heard* of it until Juliet examined me!

If you have ab separation, the core itself might not hurt, but the weakness there could lead to some serious back pain like the kind I'd been experiencing on and off since Titan arrived on the scene. I couldn't believe it! I'd thought I was so strong and taking such good care of myself, so learning that my abs were so weak so long after childbirth really threw me for a loop. Because my abs were compromised, I'd been overcompensating with my back—no wonder I was in such pain all the time! Thanks to Juliet, I could finally seek the help I needed to get better, though I'm afraid the journey might be a long one.

And surprise, surprise, I'm not the only one who's developed mysterious-seeming aches and pains after childbirth. Some women have terrible cramps; others have intense back pain. Some have pain in their joints; others have pain all over their bodies. Then again, how could we not experience some aftereffects? Pregnancy and childbirth have completely traumatized your body, so some residual pain is only to be expected. In most cases, the aches go away on their own, but by no means always, as I'm learning with my battered tailbone. If your pains are particularly bad, talk to your doctor about hooking you up with a physical therapist who can help get you back on track.

I spoke both with Juliet and with the amazing physical therapist Esther Lee about some of the most common aches and pains women have post-baby, and what you can do about them. She said in many cases these physical changes, many of which take place during pregnancy, can persist for four to six weeks after birth and may last longer if you're breastfeeding. In the majority of cases, these issues will resolve themselves, but you can also speed the process along. In my case, with the diastasis recti, the pain could linger for years before you figured out the cause. Don't wait to consult your doctor if you have a persistent physical complaint post-baby. The sooner you can work to resolve it, the faster your body will rebound.

Problem: Diastasis Recti

As I said, diastasis recti, the separation of the ab muscles, had been plaguing me for almost two years after Titan was born, and I was the last to find out about it! I thought my back pain had originated in some injury I'd sustained dancing, or during labor, when in fact the weakness had come from my core all along. And, as I learned the hard way, if your core, which holds your whole body together, is messed up, nothing works right.

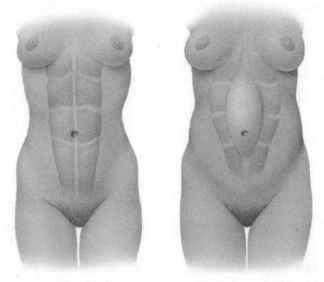

During pregnancy, the growing uterus sometimes causes the abdominal muscles to separate (diastasis recti).

IDENTIFYING—AND RECOVERING FROM— DIASTASIS RECTI

I was stunned that my abs had separated so dramatically, and I asked my new trainer, Marcela Washington, why I wasn't able to identify the problem earlier. She reassured me that many new moms are in the same boat.

"In America, if we have no complications during childbirth, we often go home the day after having a baby," Marcela told me. "Doctors probably won't look at your abdominals at the hospital, and probably won't check for diastasis recti at your six-week visit, either. Most women make the discovery that their abs have separated more informally, by sharing experiences with other women, or a midwife, or someone who happens to be part of their pregnancy. And often this happens quite some time after we've had our babies, when we're trying to understand why our bodies have changed so dramatically."

Marcela gave me some great tips on how to start tackling ab separation immediately after giving birth:

✔ **Step 1:** "Right after you've had the baby, wrap a towel around your belly close to your abdominal walls. You can use a towel, or baby blankets, or a scarf—anything that allows you to wrap the belly gently, without a lot of tension. We're all about swaddling the baby, but we need to swaddle the mommy, too!"

✔ **Step 2** (and I heard this one over and over from all the experts I consulted): "Be more aware of how you use your body, especially your core. Whether you're lifting your baby (as you'll do dozens of times a day), or getting out of bed, or rising from a chair, just pay closer attention to how you're engaging your abs. It's inevitable that you'll have lost some connection to your abs during pregnancy, so take this opportunity to support your abdominal muscles when you're going about your day."

✔ **Step 3:** "Once you're working out again, avoid exercises that push your ab muscles out—you might want to hold off on crunches, heavy weight-lifting, and even squats early on. Focus on exercises that draw your abdominal muscles inward, toward your spine, and reactivate your core. Just drawing those muscles inward not only when you exercise but when you're doing daily activities will go a long way toward knitting your abs back together."

And Marcela reminded me that, as in so much of life, prevention is the best cure. The more you've learned to strengthen those ab muscles before pregnancy, the better you'll be able to reactivate them afterward.

Solution

If your ab muscles have separated (and only a medical professional can determine this), talk to a physician, athletic trainer, or physical therapist who can customize exercises to help knit them back together. Juliet Barnes said that I had to focus on my lower abdominals rather than the general ab strengthening I'd been doing. She suggested starting with some basic pelvic tilts. I began by just lying on the floor, engaging my abs deeply, and tilting my back upward slowly while breathing deeply from my diaphragm.

"You want to make sure that you're able to move your legs while you hold the pelvic tilt posture—and you have to be able to breathe at the same time," Juliet said. When Juliet showed me the ropes, she always engaged me in conversation, distracting me with questions about what I'd eaten for lunch that day and that sort of thing. It was her way of tricking me into breathing steadily while I was doing the tilts. You also need to concentrate on keeping a neutral pelvis in everything you do, so when you're lying on the floor, your back should be flat against it, not arched upward. If your back ever begins to arch, you have to ease up on your exercises until you can keep it neutral.

Once you get the pelvic tilts down, you can move on to some more advanced exercises, like marching and doing bridges, that build on those same muscles. (Your physical therapist will help you make that progression.) And whatever your workout regimen, you should take a few minutes to lie on the floor and engage those muscles first.

Juliet said that, no matter what, I need to engage my lower abdominals three times a week while breathing deeply from my diaphragm. That kind of breathing is important for me as a singer, anyway. I'd been noticing that I'd been getting winded faster than usual in recent months, but I had *no* idea it was because of any weakness in my ab muscles!

If your ab separation is severe (as I am hoping and praying mine is not!), you might also have to wear an abdominal brace to decrease stress on your abs, and decrease back pain in the process. Surgery might ultimately be necessary, but I'm going to cross that bridge when I come to it.

Problem: Back Pain

It's a fact of life that we gain weight when we're pregnant. And more weight means more pressure on the joints, which can lead to strain, and a messed-up center of gravity, which can lead to poor posture. I was waddling around the room and not too concerned about my posture, so everything was off-kilter and imbalanced. Also, as Dr. B. explained, my ab muscles were so busy holding Titan in place that they were neglecting their usual duty of keeping me standing upright.

The surge of progesterone and relaxin in your system can also contribute to pain in both your back and your joints. When you're pregnant, you're all stretchy and loose, sometimes far more than you would be normally. After the baby's born, you add to that strain by constantly stooping over the baby—reaching down to pick him up twenty times a day, or leaning over him while nursing. (Dr. B. told me there is actually an official ailment known as "nursing neck" that occurs when you bend your neck over your baby for too long!) Most moms are so focused on their baby's comfort that they completely neglect their own.

Solutions

- Get in the habit right away of bending your knees and lifting your baby from your legs. It may seem unnecessary now, but when your forty-pound three-year-old is still demanding to be picked up every five seconds, you'll be very glad that you learned to spare your back early in the game.
- Whenever possible, try to avoid lifting the child over the top of the crib; over time, that simple action will also mess your back up in a major way. For tiny infants, you can get those raised mattresses that minimize the need to bend way down over the sleeping baby.
- Try to breastfeed while sitting fairly upright. And bring the baby toward you, rather than contorting yourself to reach him. You can try using one of those special pillows that brings the baby closer to your chest level so that you don't have to bend down as much. I know, I know—all you're

focused on is getting the baby to achieve the perfect latch, but you neglect your own body at your peril! It's possible for both you and the baby to be comfortable.

- As soon as you get cleared to exercise, go for it. Exercise has anti-inflammatory properties, and the more you move, the better your whole body will feel.
- Talk to your doctor or physical therapist about getting a belt or corset for external support.
- Modify how you perform everyday activities, like getting in and out of the car. Lying on your side with a pillow between your legs can also help.
- Try not to carry your kid on your hip; that can cause asymmetrical tension in your back muscles. Get one of those nifty baby-wearing devices so you can wear your baby right in your middle.
- Just becoming more aware of your posture will go a long way. Bend your knees and lift from your legs and try not to hunch forward too long. Try gentle stretches when you get your doctor's clearance, and go in for a massage, or just get someone you love to rub down your overworked muscles and joints. If the pain persists for more than six weeks, talk to a doctor about seeing a physical therapist.
- Losing pregnancy weight can help relieve pressure on your muscles and joints—but no rush! The weight will come off in due time if you're eating right and moving around, so don't put any additional pressure on yourself.
- A belly band won't really do much to speed up your recovery, but you might feel better when you're wearing one, especially if you've had a C-section. It might also give your

posture a lift and just hold that whole overworked area of your body together.

Problem: Cramps

You might also experience some pretty intense cramping in your abdominal region, particularly in the early days of breast-feeding. This is totally normal. It's just what your uterus contracting back to its non-baby-containing size feels like.

Solution

Good old-fashioned Tylenol can help, or you can just wait it out. The symptoms should disappear on their own within six weeks, by which point your uterus will have shrunk (mostly) back to its pre-baby size.

Problem: Pelvic Girdle Pain

Pelvic girdle pain refers to any and all pain in the pelvic region, like the type I experienced in my last few weeks of pregnancy. Your coccyx might hurt, or your lower abdomen, or your lumbar spine, and you might cringe as you walk, or climb the stairs, or lie on your side. For some women, like me, this pain is at its most intense during pregnancy; for other women, it is the act of childbirth that activates the pain.

Even if you're one of those (incredibly rare) lucky women who didn't tear, your pelvic floor has still gone through the wringer, so it's no wonder the pain lingers after childbirth. Your ligaments have gotten stretched, your tissues have gotten ripped, and your muscles have been pushed. Just take it easy on yourself so your body can do its thing.

Solutions

- Time might not heal all wounds, but it can really make a difference. Give all the overworked muscles and ligaments of your pelvis time to repair themselves. If this is something that concerns you at your six-week visit, bring it up with your doctor.
- To speed along the process, you can also lie on the floor and do pelvic tilts.
- Do Kegels! I know, I know, just what you wanted to hear. But fun or not, squeezing the muscles of your perineum over and over and over again (sigh) can really help restore the condition of your pelvis.

CRASH COURSE ON KEGELS

- Pretend you're trying to stop the flow of urine; those are the muscles you need to be activating.
- Squeeze the muscles, count to three, then release.
- Repeat fifteen times.
- Do at least four Kegel sessions per day.

- Gradually increase the time you hold until you've hit ten seconds. So on week two, hold for three seconds; on week three, hold for four.
- Consistency is key to getting the benefits of Kegels, so do them as often as you can. The best thing is that you can do them anywhere—at a stoplight, in the middle of a business lunch—and no one will be the wiser.

If sex is painful even months after your doctor has given you the green light, the problem might not be damage to your pelvis but vaginal dryness, a frequent consequence of the huge drop in estrogen levels our bodies undergo postpartum. Talk to your doctor about a topical estrogen cream that you can apply down there. If that doesn't do the trick, talk to your doctor about hooking you up with a physical therapist who can help.

Problem: All-over Achiness

Trust me, girl, I've been there. I remember that feeling so well, of every single joint and muscle just aching from deep down. My muscles would creak when I stood up and I would generally feel eighty years old whenever I got up after being in the same position for too long.

Solutions

- There's no better excuse to take a few minutes to soak in a nice warm bath—didn't you miss them when you were pregnant? They'll help ease your achy body, at least while you're submerged, and give your busy brain and body a much-needed interval of rest. Even if it's just for fifteen minutes, whenever you can, pass off your baby to another caregiver, or put the baby down (without bending too much!) for a nap, and get soaked.

- Swimming can also be a great way to exercise and stretch your body without putting any weight on tender areas.
- Try some simple yoga stretches. You can do these anywhere, anytime—but make sure you are gentle on yourself! Stretching too much can lead to as many problems as not stretching enough.
- If your pain persists beyond six weeks, talk to your medical caregiver about physical therapy. A good physical therapist can set you up with a regimen of exercises customized to your body.

PRIORITY #1:

Unlike other types of exercise, you should start doing pelvic-floor exercises immediately after delivery. They can help with incontinence, tone up the pelvic floor, and generally speed up your whole recovery process.

Problem: Prolapse

Pelvic prolapse happens when organs in your pelvic area, most commonly your uterus, fall out of place. Women who've delivered vaginally, have a history of chronic constipation or obesity, and athletes all might be at risk for this particularly un-comfortable injury, which can cause your uterus to stick down out of your vagina.

Solution

Kegels on overdrive and other pelvic-floor exercises can help stabilize your pelvic floor. Prolapse after childbirth is the result of weakened pelvic muscles, and Kegels can help strengthen them. If you think you have prolapse, you should consult your doctor or get a physical therapist recommendation. Worst-case scenarios may require surgical intervention.

General Physical Recovery Exercise Tips from Esther

- You can worry about your bikini body later; right now your priority should be to make your body whole after childbirth has traumatized it.
- Stretch, but don't stretch too much. Your joints were al-ready excessively mobile during your pregnancy. You don't want to cause damage to your joints by stretching them too much.
- Try not to stand for too long; usually not a huge problem when you're in bed with the baby for most of the day.
- Drink lots and lots of water.
- Avoid holding your breath during exercises as it may lead to increased pressure on the uterus and pelvic floor and

increased stress to the cardiovascular system, leading to increased blood pressure and heart rate.

Juliet also suggested sitting on a Swiss ball—yep, get out that old birthing ball again—to keep your ab muscles engaged throughout the day. And never forget about standing up straight; if you have good posture, you are making your abs work in the right way.

CHAPTER 15

When Can I Hit the Gym Again?

(Getting Back in Shape)

FOR THE FIRST SIX WEEKS after giving birth, doctors generally recommend refraining from exercise, and I totally get that. Your body has gone (and is going) through so much that you don't want to risk injuring yourself by overdoing it too soon. But the second Dr. Bickman gave me the all-clear to start working out again, I went right back to the gym. Because I was pretty fit when I got knocked up, I admit that I wanted—and in fact expected—to see instant results after my first day back. I was going to run five miles and do a hundred squats and basically just kick butt all around!

Boy, was I in for a rude awakening. I hopped on the treadmill, positive I was going to be just awesome even if I was still really heavy. The song "Happy" came on and that's exactly how I felt. But then, I swear within thirty seconds I was huffing and puffing and on the verge of collapse. What had happened to my cardiovascular strength that I'd spent so many years cultivating?

I was embarrassed by how little I could do. I barely made it through a single song! Once I recovered my breath, I switched to light intervals on the treadmill: a couple of alternating rounds of walking for a minute, then jogging for a minute. It was *hard*. Every time I jogged, even just for a minute, I felt like I was on the verge of having a heart attack. So, yeah, the road back to cardio was not quite as painless as I'd imagined it. Of course, not everyone has a hard time snapping back into shape. I've found that my friends who are serious runners and those who do high-intensity spinning like SoulCycle tend to bounce back faster and not get as winded as I did. Everyone's experience, at this and every other phase of the game, is totally different.

My trainer Marcela Washington had some words of wisdom for me about accepting my new body. "Be the woman that you're becoming," she told me, "because you can't go back to your old self." And, looking at Titan, I knew I didn't want to! "You're moving to something more powerful, because there's an inner strength that comes from birth. So mentally visualize the woman you're becoming, and release what you used to be."

I was also surprised by how little my return to the gym seemed to affect my waistline. I'd been panting like a fool on that treadmill; shouldn't all that extra weight just be flying off? During the six weeks right after Titan was born, I'd been sure that my inability to work out was what was really preventing me from shedding weight.

I was still too stuck in the instant-gratification mentality, but I quickly learned that that's just not how it works. Reclaiming your pre-pregnancy body doesn't happen overnight, and you can't just jump right back into some insane workout routine immediately after having a baby. Case in point: it took me an *entire year* to get back to the three-mile jog I'd been doing for years. A whole year! And I wasn't slacking off during that time. I was showing up, day in and day out, and pushing myself to my (extremely unimpressive) limits. Obviously, each woman has different challenges, and you should always consult your physician before starting to exercise again. I just wanted to share what worked to get me back on track.

KEGELS ALARM CLOCK

I just can't remind you enough. Do Kegels whenever you can. However boring they seem, they are just as important as any other exercise you might try. During those early months of working out, I would always spend a few minutes lying on the floor doing some deep breathing exercises and getting some Kegels in. Luckily, I'd gotten into the habit really early on; my incredible doula, Lori Bregman, taught me to do Kegels constantly during the pregnancy, and that preparation really helped me afterward; it was like I had no choice but to hold my vagina all damn day!

And, yes, even though it's very hard to be disciplined about Kegels, as Dr. Bickman told me, if you're not doing them ten times a day, you might as well not even bother. I kept on squeezing for the future health of my vagina. Maybe my next baby will glide right out and I won't even feel it? Yeah, I don't think so. But when you are already at the gym, or about to go out for a jog, or stream a video, or whatever it is you do to stay in shape, take a few minutes before and after to lie back and Kegel it up.

SOME EXERCISE TIPS FROM A PHYSICAL THERAPIST

- ✔ As soon as your doctor clears you, get in the habit of exercising for thirty minutes or more per day. It's better, especially early on, to focus on non-weight-bearing exercises like swimming and biking, or less strenuous exercises like walking.
- ✔ In your first weeks back in the saddle, avoid single-leg weight-bearing exercises like leg lifts. Your pelvis is still unstable and asymmetrical exercises can make it worse.
- ✔ If any exercise you attempt starts to hurt, stop! Avoid any exercises that cause discomfort or pain.
- ✔ Empty your bladder prior to initiating exercises to decrease stress on the weakened pelvic floor.
- ✔ Don't exercise to exhaustion. Your body has gone through enough recently—go easy on yourself!

—Esther Lee, DPT

The First Workout

I had one goal for my first post-baby workout: show up. When you've been out of the swing of things for so long—and when getting to the gym means separating from your baby and likely putting a hundred other obligations on hold as well—it can feel like quite an accomplishment. So if you made it, pat yourself on the back! The hard part is over. You've kissed your baby goodbye for a few minutes, you've gotten over your sadness, and you've decided to devote a few minutes to just you. That is amazing in and of itself. Even if, like me, you barely make it through a full minute of hard-core cardio, you are awesome for even lacing up those running shoes and slapping on those extra-large yoga pants. And, honestly, even if you feel as shocked as I did by how much your fitness level has gone down, try not to get too discouraged. Don't forget that your body has been fairly busy in the past year, consumed with the essential business of growing and feeding a baby.

Every workout back is an accomplishment, so again—you just have to pat yourself on the back for putting on that jogging bra and getting back in the game, or trying to. In my first several workouts, I found it really excruciatingly hard to be away from Titan. I'd feel totally unmotivated, with no desire to leave him, and also guilty, like I was squandering precious hours of his life indulging my own need to work out. It was only when I started seeing results—when I'd jump on the scale and see the numbers moving downward, or slide into a dress that hadn't fit me the week before—that my motivation became more concrete. I was finally able to say, "All right, this baby can wait for an hour. Right now is my time to take care of *me*."

Setting a Schedule

That was the next step for me: establishing a goal of how many times I wanted to work out a week—for me it was three to five times—and doing my utmost to make that goal. Consistency is *so* important. Even if I only had thirty minutes to spare, I found that I was always more energetic, and in a better mood, afterward. So it quickly became a priority for me to make the time to work out, no matter how much else I had going on. And as the weeks passed, the more I showed up, the easier it was for me to get there. Exercise has always been a powerful mood-booster for me, and I felt proud of myself for taking the time to take care of myself when I was spending so much of myself taking care of Titan. When we're giving so much of our bodies and minds over to nurturing the people we love (especially the tiniest ones), we need to make even more of an effort to nurture ourselves, too. I wanted to be a strong mother both inside and out, so I kept having to remind myself that the better shape I was in, the better I could take care of the people I loved. Once I'd set my schedule, I was ready to begin.

Stage 1: Cardio

In the beginning, for my first two weeks back, I just did cardio—that's it. Get that heart rate up and call it a day. I totally stayed away from the hot mess that was my abdominal region in those early weeks. Instead I just got back on the treadmill and started the slow, slow process of building up my endurance again.

But even though I didn't do core exercises, I did try to engage my core right out of the gate. If I was jogging at my snail's pace, then I was pulling in my navel. If I was lying on the floor doing Kegels, I was pulling in my navel. Whatever I did, I tried to keep that core awake and engaged.

When you have a baby wedged in your abdomen for the better part of a year, you can be forgiven for losing your connection with that whole region of your body. You've given your abs over to the growing baby inside, and afterward you have a lot of catch-up work to do.

Constantly pulling in your ab muscles, no matter what you're doing, will help you avoid (or reverse) that diastasis recti. So even when I was walking across the room to get Titan, I was engaging more muscles all over my body by making a conscious effort to pull my navel to my spine. And, after a while, the effort became less conscious and I just did it automatically.

Here's a trick to make sure you're pulling your navel toward your spine and pulling the belly in flat. Try wrapping a towel around the back of your torso and pulling it upward, tight around your navel, as you crunch. Not everyone has a trainer, obviously, so the towel really helps you to physically feel what's going on in your abs. It slows you down and forces you to think about pulling your navel toward your spine. When you crunch up, you're pulling the towel from each side up toward the center of your body, an action that serves as a reminder to you to pull in your navel.

One more embarrassing admission. In addition to being shockingly out of shape, I also seemed to get a little, er, "gassy" (that is my polite southern term for "farting a lot") during my postpartum workouts. Dr. Bickman told me that it was probably because the pelvic muscles that usually control these activities had gotten all stretched and loose. I tried not to be too embarrassed about these little interruptions, reminding myself that all new moms, including the most put-together-looking ones, can toot without warning post-baby.

Stage 2: Core Strength Training

Once I could get through a few consecutive minutes of jogging without turning purple and wanting to pass out, I progressed to the next stage, which was strength training, particularly in the abdominal area. At the time, of course, I didn't yet know about my diastasis recti. If I had, I probably would've done less to "get in shape" and more to heal; that is, wrapping my belly in a towel like Marcela suggested and doing some restorative pelvic tilts right out of the gate.

As it was, I mixed it up a lot, always returning to the cardio: a little bit of cardio, a little bit of light weight-lifting, a little bit of cardio, a little bit of yoga and Pilates exercises. I did lots of planks and lots of Kegels and I always, always pulled in my navel so that my flapping abs at least *looked* flatter.

My mom once said to me, "My tummy was never the same after you were born!" But I'm not down with that kind of fatalistic thinking. Don't blame it on the baby—just go work out! If you keep your core engaged in everything you do, your entire body will recover faster, even if, as I learned with my abdominal separation, it can take quite a few years to fix. It's all about the core. Your baby did quite a number on that part of the body, but you *can* get your strength back there. It just might not be an overnight fix.

Stage 3: The Whole Package

Into my second month of working out again, I continued to focus on my poor, beat-up abs. It was only once I felt like all my sucking-in had finally woken up that part of my body again that I started to get into a modified version of what I'd done pre-baby. For me, that meant jogging and strength training with some yoga and Pilates mixed in. Whatever you did before baby, you can start doing again in earnest about six weeks after you've started exercising again.

The length of my workouts depended on what I had going on that day, but I generally tried to do at least thirty minutes, a full hour if I was feeling particularly motivated. (But whatever you can fit in is better than nothing, so even if you have just fifteen minutes to do some ab exercises, your body will thank you for it.) I'd generally do twenty to thirty minutes of cardio, then some strength training, whether that meant planks or some Pilates or yoga or some work with free weights. I always like to mix it up a little, but the basic order of operations was the same—kick it off with cardio, then follow it up with strength training.

WHAT EXERCISE CAN FIX

Exercise isn't a cure-all, and you can't expect your body to return to its previous shape instantaneously, or ever, even with lots of effort. Even now, when I'm totally happy with my weight and my body, I feel like staying in shape requires more work than it did before. That's why it's so helpful for me to remember all the ways exercise feeds my body and spirit. It can:

- Boost your energy levels, which is more important than ever now that you've added that sweet little baby to your daily juggle.

- Tighten your skin. This was important to me post-baby because I just could not deal with that sheet of flab hanging off my abdomen.

Lifting heavier weights can create more tone in the muscles and more tension in the skin, which helps obliterate that loose skin you get after pregnancy. (Making sure you're eating healthy and getting the proper nutrients, particularly protein, is also important for skin elasticity.) Heavy weight-training helps tone everything: your butt, your back, your abs, all of it.

- Help shed the pounds. There are so, so many factors to losing weight (not to mention keeping it off), and a regular exercise regimen is definitely high on the list. Obviously your diet and your genes play a huge role as well, but exercise is a big component in getting your body back to its dream dimensions.

- Maintain your sanity. Exercise gives you the now-more-necessary-than-ever opportunity to step back, calm down, and just focus on *you* for a change. Whether it's for twenty minutes or an hour a day, however many times a week you can squeeze it in, your workout will give you mental clarity, which is just as important as all the physical benefits.

As you embark on this journey, don't make the mistake I did and expect an overnight transformation. No matter how hard you work, your body has gone through a great deal, so go easy on it. Even though I was incredibly disciplined about working out, I'd say it took me all of ten or eleven months to start feeling like myself again. By Titan's first birthday, I was about five pounds heavier than I'd been pre-baby, but that seemed like a small price to pay for my little nugget.

Just as I'd started to accept my new weight, I took a ballet class, and you'll never believe what happened—I lost eight more pounds! So by the time Titan was eighteen months old, I weighed slightly less than I did pre-pregnancy, and I have to say that felt amazing. But I truly believe that the reason I was able to get back down to my regular weight was because I let go of my perfectionism and just let my body do its own thing on its own time line (and did some ballet!).

CHAPTER 16

How Am I Supposed to Do This?

(Insecurity)

WITH SO MANY OF US first-time moms, the perfectionism doesn't end at the gym. So many of us pregnant newbies are so, so excited to give birth, but then we get home and realize that we have no clue what we are doing. You can feel like an impostor—like this person playacting at being a good mom when deep down you have absolutely no clue what you're doing.

These feelings of insecurity seem inevitable when everyone in your life seems to have the whole motherhood thing totally down: former classmates you're friends with on Facebook, women in line in front of you at Target, and especially all the perfectly coiffed celebrities splashed across every magazine cover.

Meanwhile, you are totally exhausted and overwhelmed and barely keeping it together, and you feel even worse when you compare yourself to all those other competent-looking parents around you.

News flash for you. You're not the only mom who has ever felt this way, and there's absolutely nothing wrong with you.

I've said it before and I'll say it again: Your tiny infant is not going to remember if you didn't change his diaper the very second he wet it. He's not going to remember if you didn't pick him up the first second he cried or if you left him in the crib for a few more minutes while you took a shower. You might remember it, but your baby won't. Babies might seem fragile, but in fact they're incredibly resilient, so you can screw up all you want (within reason, of course), and your baby won't hold it against you.

In fact, there might be something wrong with you if you *didn't* feel this way. That's because none of us have a clue what we're doing the first time we become parents. It doesn't matter if you're the oldest of eight children or have never laid eyes on a newborn before—having your own baby is a whole new ballgame that comes with a whole new set of rules. Unfortunately, no one tells you those rules, so you have to make them up as you go along. But we're all in the same boat!

One of the most helpful things a girlfriend told me when I was expecting was that we don't get a manual for parenting; it's all about on-the-job training. So much of this you just learn as you go. Every parent is different, and so is every child, so you can read all the books and scribble down all the advice you want, but you're not going to know what to do until you've got that baby in your arms. And even then you still might not know—and that's totally okay!

If you're used to excelling at work, or being a totally amazing wife, or just generally being awesome at whatever you're doing at any given time, you need to put that Type A streak to rest for a while. Parenting is not a race or a competition. We are all just doing the best we can with what we've been given, and we're all under enough pressure without setting ourselves up with unreasonable expectations. Just keep reminding yourself that none of us really know what we're doing, and the best solution is to band together and help one another out. There is no such thing as a perfect parent or a perfect child or the perfect way of doing something. It's all just trial and error.

The more you do it, the more you know, and the more you know, the less afraid you are of screwing up or not measuring up to your peers. And, by the way, if your friends tell you that they lost all the weight in two weeks, or got their kids to sleep through the night at two months, or whatever it is that is making you feel insecure, then remind yourself that they're probably lying. And even if they're not, then they'll get their turn to go through the wringer with their kids. Maybe your friend who has the easiest infant will wake up one day to the most stubborn toddler, or the sweet-natured toddler will become the most mule-headed tween. No kid is easy 100 percent of the time.

So the version you are getting in your friend's perfect Facebook feeds is not the whole story, not even close. We're in this cultural moment where we are putting filters on every part of our lives, but there's no filter for parenthood, for what it's like to actually have a child. You can try to make it look prettier all you want, but you won't be fooling any of us who've been through the gauntlet—you'll just be making everyone else feel bad.

CHAPTER 17

Why Can't I Stop Crying?

(Postpartum Depression)

Now THAT I'VE TALKED so much about what the female body goes through in the process of giving birth, I want to shift from the physical side of things to the equally massive changes we undergo in our emotional lives. I just want to say it straight out. Sometimes after you give birth you can get really, really depressed. While it may seem strange to feel down about bringing new life into the world, it's actually completely normal, not that you'd know it from how little we talk about it in our society.

A huge number of women—as in, well, more than half of them—get what's known as the "baby blues," the least severe form of depression associated with childbirth. You may recognize the symptoms: you're teary for no reason you can name, you're irritable, you're completely anxious, you're impatient, you might feel like you don't even know who you are anymore. One big explanation for these unpredictable emotions is the combination of exhaustion and wildly fluctuating hormones and, as both your sleep schedule and hormone levels normalize, you'll likely feel much more stable within two or three weeks.

DIFFERENTIATING BETWEEN
NORMAL EMOTIONAL SWINGS AND RED FLAGS

One of the most important things that therapist Joe Bolduc and I discussed throughout my pregnancy, and after Titan's birth, was the impact of hormonal changes on your emotions. It's totally normal to experience big emotional swings during pregnancy and in the postpartum period, and I certainly had my share of crying-during-TV-commercial moments, and feeling generally overwhelmed. Most of the time, these emotional swings are expected and normal; nothing to worry about. But for some women, particularly those with a history of depression, anxiety, or obsessive compulsive disorder, the surge of emotions can create "red flag" emotionality that could signal developing depression or anxiety.

Some women are afraid of bringing up these red flags to their physicians. Don't be. These are issues that doctors should be trained to address. You might also want to find what Joe and I call a "pregnancy ally" during this time: a trusted friend you can feel safe sharing your emotions with—no matter how silly or outrageous—and who will speak up if you begin to exhibit any concerning moods or behaviors. You should never feel ashamed of what you suspect might be postpartum depression and anxiety; the very worst thing you can do is keep it to yourself. So whatever you do, tell someone.

But what happens if you *don't* feel more stable after the first few weeks? What happens if you don't "just get over it"? The far more serious mood disorder known as postpartum depression is scarily common—as many as *one in seven* new mothers experience it—but somehow it's a totally untouchable subject.

The fact that we talk so little about postpartum depression seems even more tragic when you really crunch the numbers. If approximately 4 million babies are born in the United States every year and one out of every seven of their mothers has postpartum depression, that's 570,000 women we're talking about!

But somehow we just don't hear about this serious disorder nearly enough, and hundreds of thousands of women continue to suffer in silence needlessly. And, as we're learning, so do their babies, since maternal stress, depression, and anxiety are all too easily transmitted to the baby.

My dear friend Joe Bolduc, a therapist who has worked with a lot of women struggling with depression at the onset of motherhood, explained to me that the huge hormonal surge brought on by pregnancy and childbirth can really activate mental illnesses and depressions and anxieties, or obsessive compulsive disorders that have been dormant. That means that if you have a history of anxiety or depression, you might be more at risk for having postpartum depression. So, please, if you fall into this category, just be on the lookout, and have your loved ones monitor you for unusual emotions during and after your pregnancy. And no matter what, never ever hesitate to ask for help.

Because—this is the message we need to be repeating over and over again—it's not "just in your head." Postpartum depression is a very real illness that requires very real intervention. As I spoke to friends and mothers while researching this book, I was completely amazed—and not in a good way—by how little support there is out there, and how little knowledge. Instead there's just a lot of shame and misinformation.

But given the effects of depression, we simply can't afford to allow so many women to suffer in silence. We need to start investing much more time and resources in educating women to recognize the signs of postpartum depression and other mental illnesses, and we also need to offer more avenues of treatment.

Let me say this. If your "baby blues" last more than a couple of weeks, if you feel detached from or unable to take care of your infant and find yourself crying for no reason, see your doctor ASAP. There are medical professionals out there who can support you through this hugely rewarding—but also hugely difficult—transition, and if you think you might be depressed after having a baby, do not hesitate to get yourself the care you need right away. Call your doctor. Call the hospital where you delivered. Getting help doesn't have to be expensive; the hospital will be able to connect you with free resources and counseling that are available in many communities. The hardest part is the first step of acknowledging that you need help. But I promise once you get there, you'll find a tremendous number of people who want nothing more than to help you through to the other side.

WHY IT MATTERS

There's finally serious, in-depth research being done on postpartum depression, and what we're learning is that women who suffer from depression and anxiety have through-the-roof levels of the stress hormone cortisol, which can affect the mother's internal organs—her liver, her heart, her central nervous system. All of it goes into the baby. We're finding that babies of women who are depressed and anxious are being born with high, high levels of cortisol, so they're starting off their lives with stressors. These babies can be harder to soothe, more colicky, and more environmentally sensitive than other babies, and that can create a feedback loop. You've got this colicky baby who's hard to soothe, and cranky and unhappy, with a depressed mother who is having a hard time dealing with it anyway. Later on, these children might wind up with developmental issues, or problem behaviors, or anxiety, or attachment issues. Babies are incredibly perceptive, and if their mothers are suffering, they're going to pick up on that on some level.

We need to really start looking at postpartum depression from a societal perspective. We need to value women's pregnancies because we're going to be dealing with their babies as grown-ups. It all starts by teaching women to become more aware of their emotions as they navigate this complicated time.

—Joe Bolduc

I was lucky enough not to experience postpartum depression; when Titan arrived on the scene, despite everything that was going on with my body, I was just in total happy bliss.

But I did undergo a major trauma when Titan was just three weeks old that taught me about how unpredictable life can be, and how the best and the worst events always seem to pile up at the same time. What happened was that my mother, Doris Garrison, died suddenly and completely unexpectedly. She'd been there when I gave birth, and three weeks later she was gone.

When I got the out-of-the-blue call that she'd gone into cardiac arrest, I didn't even know how to process it. My immediate thought was that of course nothing bad was going to happen to her. "Doris always pulls through everything," I told myself. "She'll come out of this just fine." My whole life, she'd always been such a fighter—why should this time be any different?

Even though it was December, right in the middle of flu season, and I was totally petrified to fly with a newborn, Titan and I boarded a plane and flew across the country to Atlanta. When we got there, my mom was already brain dead. I just couldn't believe it. When I walked into the hospital room and saw her hooked up to a million tubes, with all those monitors flashing, the reality of what was happening hit me for the first time. "Oh, shit, I'm about to lose my mom," I thought.

Letting her go came as a huge, horrible shock, but part of me was still so focused on Titan's well-being that I really didn't give myself the opportunity to plunge into the deep sadness I would've felt even a month earlier. The necessity of devoting so much of my energy and emotions to my baby turned out to be an incredibly powerful healing tool for me.

If I ever felt like I was about to cry, I would have Tim or one of his aunts take over for a few minutes, and I'd go to a room and cry by myself. I wouldn't do it in front of Titan—I just did not want to pass any of my sorrow on to him. So instead I would sit by myself and pray and let myself be sad for as long as I needed to. Then, slowly, I would try to bring myself out of it by thinking about his birth and picturing his sweet little face. That was how, even without being in the room with me, my baby would bring me light, and I'd start to feel happy again.

The name Titan means "one who is strong," and I felt in those moments that God had sent me a Titan to bring me strength and heal my heart at a time when I needed it most. My

I can't tell you the number of first-time moms who, even without a family tragedy, call me in distress a few days after they've come home with their new baby. "This is so crazy and overwhelming," they'll cry. "No one ever told me it was going to be like this! I'm not going to make it!" I assure them that, no matter how hard it seems at first, they won't always feel this way. When I tell patients that what they're going through is normal, they usually say something like, "Oh my God, *really*?" This reaction isn't all that surprising when you consider how little information there is out there about how hard those first weeks are.

Then, six weeks later, they bounce into my office a totally new person. The baby isn't screaming and waking up so much, they're getting a little more sleep, they've adjusted to nursing, they're no longer in such acute pain. They might even be wearing makeup again!

No matter how unbelievable it may seem when you have a teeny-tiny, around-the-clock-needy newborn, things usually will turn around for you at six to eight weeks. By three months you'll feel even better, and by a year you will (mostly) have adapted to your crazy new life. Of course, if a patient has a history of depression or is experiencing some unusual psychiatric symptoms, I will immediately refer her to a psychiatrist, but this is actually pretty rare.

intense connection to my baby helped me get through what was one of the hardest experiences of my life. I swear I'm not putting sauce on this situation after the fact; it's just honestly how I felt, then and now. My faith—which my mother instilled in me, and which I now think of as a gift she left me—took over, and I was able to let go of some of the challenges we'd had in the past and focus on all the wonderful things she taught me, all the different ways she prepared me to become a good mother.

Still, losing my mom was a huge, huge trauma to process when I was still adjusting to motherhood, when so much of my life was totally new and unknown, and somehow, for all the support they lent me, even my closest friends had trouble asking me about my feelings during this time. And it made me understand the extent to which having a baby intensifies all your emotions, good and bad. Even without postpartum depression, feeling psychotically tired can make you lose perspective. You're already dealing with your body changing, your whole dynamic changing—how do you make those adjustments mentally? I had so many questions that Joe and I would discuss at length.

I want to share in the next chapter some of the advice Joe offered me, which I believe can be of tremendous service to new mothers regardless of their circumstances, or mental and emotional situation. The key, Joe taught me, is to start the process during pregnancy, so that you're in a stronger place after the baby shows up, when you're at your most emotionally vulnerable.

I honestly believe the self-examination I did while pregnant helped me weather the shock of losing my mom. With Joe's guidance I got myself ready, while Titan was still in my body, for the changes motherhood would bring, and those measures were crucial in laying the groundwork for how I handled the transition afterward.

CHAPTER 18

What Do I Want Out of Motherhood?

(Getting Your Brain Ready)

WHEN I TALKED TO Joe Bolduc during the weeks leading up to Titan's birth, he kept encouraging me to examine my life and situation more deeply so that I'd be on solid ground when the baby showed up and turned my world upside down forevermore. "What happens postpartum gets planned while you're pregnant," he kept telling me, and that became my mantra as I began to contemplate some of the most fundamental things in my life.

I didn't want parenthood to be something that just happened to me. I wanted to play an active role in shaping my, and my future baby's, experience well before I even became a mother. I wanted to feel actionable in the changes coming to my life, and that's something every single woman can do, no matter what their career or relationship or romantic situation. Of course, postpartum depression is not something you can plan your way around, but I think examining your state of mind before you give birth can serve as a good signpost if something goes wrong afterward. Whether you're single and the pregnancy was unplanned, or whether you've been trying for a baby for years, you can set yourself up for a positive experience of motherhood by really thinking out your state of mind in the present moment and articulating your dreams for the future.

It all starts by asking yourself some tough questions and really examining what type of mother you want to become. You have so much more control than you realize. No matter who you are, you can shape your experience of pregnancy and motherhood. Not only can you shape it, you *must* shape it.

Step 1: Examine your own childhood (for better or worse).

One of the most valuable things Joe had me do during my pregnancy, which I really recommend all women try, was to take the time to sit down and really think through my own childhood, and try to put my finger on what went right and what went wrong. Even before my mom's death, I'd really devoted myself to reflecting on our relationship, and it became very clear to me, when thinking over the choices she made, that nobody gets a "How to Be a Mother" book. You don't get a whole detailed instruction guide the way you would if you bought a frigging blender. We're all just figuring it out as we go along, on the fly, and that's exactly what my mom did.

My mom was wonderful and loving in so many ways, but she also led a really chaotic life, and so my life as a child was also marked by a lot of chaos. We moved a lot, and my dad wasn't really in the picture, and from that I learned that I don't thrive amid chaos, and I didn't want my future children to grow up like that. My mom was a nanny when I was growing up, so I was able to get a glimpse of another way of life, of the jobs and the people she worked for and the type of households they had, so even as a kid I knew I wanted that kind of life for my future children.

It was by thinking over my own childhood that I realized how important it was for me to be able to provide my child with a stable, peaceful household and a great father. And of course I knew that I wanted to be a great mother (whatever that meant!) as well, because I understood that Tim and I would be Titan's first role models. I grew up with a lot of different fears, but I wanted Titan and any future children I might have to grow up completely fearless. I wanted Titan to feel like he could be great at anything he put his mind to. I wanted him to feel like he could fly.

Step 2: Ask yourself some big questions.

Once I'd confronted my own past, I was able to get into more detail about my future goals as a parent. Joe prodded me to ask some pretty big questions about my dreams and goals, both for Titan and for myself. Sometimes it's the most basic-seeming questions that most get to the heart of the matter: What do you want? What kind of pregnancy do you want? What kind of mother do you want to be? What kind of mother do you not want to be? What does it mean to be a good mother? What scares you the most about being a mother? What excites you the most? In the process of going down this list of questions and attempting to answer them as honestly as possible, I came to think really hard about what I wanted and how I was going to get there.

THE GOOD-MOTHER EXERCISE

One day, Joe asked me to name any person, real or fictional, I considered an "ideal mother." Without hesitating, I named Clair Huxtable from *The Cosby Show*. Then Joe had me write down the qualities that had always made Mrs. Huxtable seem like the perfect mom to me. The way she effortlessly seemed to juggle a high-powered career with a big household of kids; the way she was firm but fair; the way she could be both a friend and a guide; her stable marriage; the secure home she helped provide for her family. I tried to keep those qualities in the front of my mind as I considered my own circumstances and how they did and did not differ from Clair's. Obviously Clair Huxtable was a TV character and real life is far messier, but I found it useful to write down what exactly made me admire her so much when I was a kid, and what about her TV persona I wanted to emulate in my own parenting.

From there, I started getting into even deeper questions: Who *am* I? Who else is telling me what I'm supposed to be? Who do *I* want to be? What is this career? What do I want it to be? What do I want to say? And on and on—it never really ends if you let yourself really get into it. In some ways, I felt like my pregnancy provided me with the first opportunity in my entire life to really look at myself and where I'd been and where I wanted to go. I think all women can take this moment to examine their lives without fear or shame. Regardless of your circumstances, you're creating a life, and that's a pretty amazing accomplishment. Never forget the miracle of that. Whether you're a pregnant teenager or you've been married twenty years, you are completely amazing for growing a new life inside you.

Step 3: Check in with yourself.

Doing constant check-ins with yourself, not just postpartum but while you're pregnant, is an important tool for figuring out if you might be depressed. And learning to get in touch with your emotions will serve you well throughout your whole life as a parent.

How are you feeling today? How off your baseline are you? Should you talk to someone? When you're pregnant and *especially* once you've had your baby, you will understandably go through a huge roller coaster of emotions. Your whole body has been hijacked, and your identity has changed forever. But what is just fatigue and "being hormonal," and what is depression that you need to pay attention to? What does depression look like?

Women often feel guilty about having negative thoughts during and after pregnancy, and all the more so because they think that no other woman has ever entertained them before. But if we do a better job of acknowledging the reality of depression, women might be more willing to step back and try to identify the difference between being tired and overwhelmed and being in a potentially dangerous place. Our society teaches us that pregnancy and motherhood should be all joy all the time, but anyone who's experienced it firsthand knows just how reductive that can be.

The downside of our society's tendency to idealize pregnancy and motherhood is that women who aren't feeling entirely positive can feel even more alienated. What if you're having a baby on your own? What if you have no money? What if you feel too young or too old for motherhood? What if you just feel inadequate? In those cases, it's even more important for you to be constantly checking in with your state of mind so that you can differentiate between the normal and not-so-normal emotions.

But of course, none of this means that you're "supposed" to feel one way or another when your child is born. You also need to accept that, at every step in this process, your feelings might be totally different from what you expected them to be, or even from what they were the previous day.

We tell women that motherhood is supposed to be this spiritually transcendent experience right from the very first second they lay eyes on their baby, and that's just not the case for everyone. It could take you days or even weeks to bond with your baby—it's a huge adjustment that all women process differently. There's nothing wrong with you if you don't instantaneously have the reaction you think you should have. Again, it's all about checking in with your feelings at every step along the way, monitoring yourself to determine if what you *are* feeling, whether it conforms to the storybook fantasy or not, is healthy or potentially problematic.

Step 4: Draw new boundaries.

To keep my state of mind free and clean, I also tried to draw new boundaries in my relationships during my pregnancy, and that meant being more honest both with myself and with the people around me about what I needed at that time of my life. And part of that was learning to say no sometimes, to become less afraid of disappointing people. I had this one girlfriend who was going through a lot of personal tumult during my pregnancy. Every time I spoke to her, she had some new terrible story to share, which she did in great detail. While of course I wanted to be there for her, at one point I just said to myself, "Having these conversations is really stressing me out, and I don't want this for my kid." Joe had told me about how higher cortisol levels in my system could affect the baby, so I really wanted to feel more peace in my life, which meant limiting the number of interactions I had that caused me stress or anxiety.

So, with respect to my friend, I made the difficult decision to draw an invisible line between us. I didn't stop talking to her altogether, of course, but instead of answering the phone every single time she called (and she called a *lot*), I'd sometimes text her back instead. "Hey, what's up," I'd write, and then I'd get the edited version. When I did pick up the phone, I'd sometimes cut her off early in the conversation and say, "You know what? I'm going to change the energy of this call and I'm going to be the thermometer. I'm not going to allow your temperature to completely change the rest of my day or my thinking."

To my surprise, she totally got where I was coming from and she seemed fine no longer off-loading all of her personal tumult on me. My decision also in a way made our friend-ship more substantive when we weren't exclusively running through the daily soap opera of her life at that time. Whenever I felt guilty for not talking to her as often as I used to, I had to stop and reprogram myself and just say, "Kelly, you did what you needed to do for yourself and for the baby and for the peace of your home."

I made even more radical changes with people less close to me. With Joe's help, I tried to distance myself from anyone who seemed toxic, or manipulative, or aggressive. Sad to say it, but we all have people in our lives who fall into this category: the energy suckers, the emotional vampires who take and take and take and never seem to have anything to give in return. For the first time in my life, I was okay saying, "Sorry, no, I'm not giving you money. No, I can't get you a job. I need to focus on me right now. I'm pregnant and I just can't do this right now. No, you can't come here for a month. No, you can't come for two weeks, or even for three days. Now is just not a good time for me." I started learning to say no when I was pregnant, and after I had Titan I found even more courage just to draw boundaries. As every mom knows, we are always pulled in so many directions in our lives, so it's helpful if you can learn to say, "Thanks, but right now I am putting my peace of mind and my baby first."

So whatever your situation—maybe you're a single mom and you've got people in your life who are shaming you, who are undermining you during (or about) your pregnancy, or who are just sucking too much life out of you—you need to feel very comfortable, not just for your sake but for the health of the baby, about disengaging. You're on the verge of creating a brand-new story for yourself and your baby, and it's okay if you tweak the cast of characters in it.

MAKING AN INVENTORY

"I have all of my clients, especially those going through a huge transition like pregnancy, take an honest inventory of the people in their life," Joe told me. "I literally have them get out a pen and write down all the people in their life, and then, next to each person's name, I have them write the percentage those people give versus the percentage they get. How much of a drain versus how much support is this person? Who are the people that are sabotaging you? Who are the people that are toxic? When you're done, look at that inventory and focus on the names of those people who take a lot and don't give much. I'm not saying you have to eliminate them from your life, but I do encourage you to spend more time with the people in the other column, the ones who fill you up. Invite them into your life and be deliberate about it. Often, people find writing these inventories to be revelatory, and you might discover that you approach some of your relationships differently afterward."

Step 5: Find your support network.

The other side of the coin is to seek out people who strengthen you. If possible, as soon as you find out you're pregnant, start getting your support network together. Who are the people around you that are going to help you and make this a better experience? Who can help support you in this miraculous experience? Is your mother a pillar of strength for you, or is she constantly talking down to you? Who are the support systems in your world? Have you put in place the people who can support you so that you can have the best relationship you can have with your baby? Lay the foundations now. This is particularly important if you're going it alone, but all moms can benefit from reconnecting. Even if you've lost touch with an old friend who is now at a similar life phase, take this opportunity to reach out and reestablish bonds with that friend. Don't wait.

And I'm not just talking about family and friends; it's also important for you to seek out a more formal support network. Be proactive. Start calling hospitals, so that when the baby comes you can get experts to do home visits with you—you would be shocked by how many hospitals offer this service for free. Look into parents' Listservs in your neighborhood and find out if there are any convenient mommy-and-me groups nearby. Again, these are incredibly common even outside of big cities.

Having a group of women with children roughly the same age as yours can be incredibly helpful for you as you navigate the sleepless nights and the teething and the ear infections and all the other dramas that come along during your first year of parenting. (These meetups also give you a chance to get out of the house every once in a while, which can be essential during those sometimes isolating months of maternity leave.) You need a village of moms who are in the trenches at the same time to help you get through the tough moments. Find people who've done it before, and people who are doing it for the first time right alongside you. We're each other's own best resources!

My girlfriends who've just had babies now call me literally every single day with questions they don't feel comfortable asking anyone else. A friend with a four-week-old called me just yesterday to ask if her boobs would ever go back to normal. I said, "Hell no!" She then asked me if her vajayjay would ever be tight again. I said, "Relax, you just pushed a baby out!" She said, yes, but does it change, does it ever go back to what it was before? She had a million questions—and that was just one of the many I had that I could never have imagined before I became a mom. It was a nice reminder that we're all in this together, and we're all learning as we go along. It really helps if you have friends on the journey with you.

Step 6: Use your pregnancy as a tool for personal transformation.

As I prepared myself mentally for Titan, I found that something else was going on. I was becoming a new person. Motherhood is a kind of birth not just for the child but for the person giving birth. You are changed forever, in every conceivable way. That can be frightening, or it can be exhilarating. I decided to go for Option #2. I wanted to push myself in new directions, both personally and professionally. Your life is going to change forever no matter what; why not use this as an opportunity to grow in all sorts of different directions?

With that goal in mind, I continued to ask myself some tough questions: Where am I now, and where am I going next? How can I value myself and my pregnancy and, by extension, my baby? How can I shape this incredible experience and make it truly my own? And how can I take care of myself so that I can do a better job of taking care of my baby?

This last question is key. As you're on the verge of becoming a caretaker, you can't neglect yourself along the way. So no matter how overwhelmed you are, or how much you've got going on, you *have* to get into the early habit of taking time out just for you—yes, even on those days when getting in a shower seems like a major accomplishment. Time will become a much more precious commodity when your baby shows up, so be very deliberate about how you use it. Take yourself seriously, and at the same time, go easier on yourself. Try to forgive yourself for what you inevitably fail to do exactly right as a parent. Appreciate what's special in the present moment even if your circumstances aren't ideal. Basically, it all boils down to honoring yourself however you can, and that can be as simple as taking a few minutes entirely to yourself every single day.

CREATING YOUR SACRED SPACE

Every single day, whether I was traveling or recording or just trying to work the breast pump, I tried to take ten minutes just to myself. It doesn't sound like much, but it can make all the difference between feeling frazzled and being truly present. Even that short amount of time can change your hormone and stress levels. I personally started meditating more and more in the year after Titan was born. I tried a lot of different apps, like Headspace, Mindfulness, and Insight Timer—there are tons to choose from out there—and found that just sitting quietly with myself for a few minutes a day really helped me face everything else that was going on around me.

So ask yourself, "How do I find my peace?" Is it by meditating, or listening to a favorite song, or dancing, or doing some yoga? Whatever it is, find a space to do it, and dedicate a time every single day to get quiet with yourself and tap into that happiness. It's a way of honoring yourself and your experience. No matter what you've got going on, you deserve ten minutes all to yourself every day—and never forget that investing in yourself is investing in the infant.

Motherhood was also a springboard for me to become braver, and not just when it came to cutting off unhealthy relationships, but when it came to making decisions in my professional life. Motherhood put the things that used to scare me in perspective. When it came to professional risks, I always used to ask myself, "What if they say no?" But for whatever reason, the question now shifted to "Well, shit, what if they say yes? Why not try?" My gran-gran used to tell me, "If you didn't try, you failed," and I finally understood what she meant by that. What's the worst that can happen, someone says no? Who cares? Then try something else. It's a whole new world out there. You're a mom now. You can be a whole new you.

CHAPTER 19

Why Can't I Relate to My Partner Anymore?

("Diamonds or Dishes")

FOR BETTER OR WORSE, something happens when you and your partner have baby number one. You stop being just a couple and start being a family. And while that transformation is 90 percent wonderful and amazing, it's definitely not seamless. I know some couples have had serious relationship issues post-baby because the mom has felt resentful and the dad has felt helpless, or just because both of them are too exhausted to make time for their relationship. But like everything in this crazy period, the bumps are temporary if you acknowledge them and take the time to work through them.

I have to confess that Tim and I really didn't have the post-baby relationship hurdles that so many people have experienced. If anything, becoming parents brought us closer together than before, with a few exceptions early on that I will discuss in the next chapter on sex. Tim was obsessed with the baby from the second he was born (well, from the second we found out I was pregnant, actually), and that totally turned me on. It was like he was the only other person in the universe who fully understood just how big a deal our baby was, and that's exactly how it should be.

In the weeks that followed Titan's birth, Tim's total devotion to the baby kept growing stronger with every second. Whenever I watched Tim play with Titan and look at him with total adoration, I really felt like I must've done something right in my life to receive such a perfect gift—both the baby and the man. And when Titan got a little older and could respond more to his daddy's adoration, well, that was even better. The smile that lit up my boy's face when his daddy walked into the room just killed me! Still does. Seeing that deep connection they shared made me feel even more connected to both of them, if that was even possible.

But trust me, I know how lucky I am to have such a supportive man on the scene. I've spoken to many friends who've had the opposite experience and felt totally alienated from their partners in those first weeks of their child's life. One told me that, after the baby, everything her husband did—or didn't do—around the house annoyed the crap out of her. Why couldn't he empty the dishwasher without being told? Could he really just breeze right by that huge mountain of laundry in the hallway and not think, "Hey, maybe I'll throw that in the washing machine"? She even got annoyed when he put his hand on her hip, because how could he possibly even be *thinking* about physical affection at a time when her body was so completely battered and drained?

And, yes, I totally get it. You can't have sex yet (and honestly it's probably the last thing on your mind), you no longer have the time just to chill out together because you're so busy with (and consumed by) the baby, you can barely finish a sentence before getting interrupted by some really pressing infant emergency. You're barely sleeping and constantly on the verge of passing out with exhaustion, your body looks like total you-know-what, and your husband, whose six-pack is still intact, breezes in all refreshed from the gym or some fun business lunch looking as fine as ever.

Of course, you're the mom, you're the one who carried the baby, and if you're breastfeeding you're the one responsible for feeding it, so there's only so much your partner can do, no matter how helpful or devoted he or she is. That's not a reason to get angry; that's just how it is.

When I talked to Dr. Bickman about all the trouble women have getting their relationships back on track post-baby, she had a great solution for me. Either you get your wife some diamonds (or whatever push present she has her heart set on) or you help out with the dishes, or some combination of the above.

Because, sure, expensive jewelry is great, but so is helping out around the house. "If you can't do the diamonds," Dr. Bickman says, "then do the dishes. You'd be surprised how grateful your partner will be for some extra help. The important, essential thing is that you just do something, *anything*, to make life easier for her in those rocky first weeks."

For me, even when Tim said something hilarious or just acknowledged that what I was doing was legit exhausting made a huge difference for me. Anything you do, big or small, to

remind the person who just gave birth that she has a committed partner in this whole endeavor will pay off in the overall life
of your relationship. The partner who didn't give birth gets off
pretty easy in this phase, but that doesn't mean the scales have
to be totally tipped. Everyone can make a contribution.

As for you, new mama, try to think of your partner's feelings,
too. It's a tremendous change for both of you, and sometimes
it's the partners who didn't give birth who can feel the most
disconnected or displaced. And it makes sense, right? It's like
this tiny little creature has taken their woman away from them,
and they have to compete for affection for the first time. However crazy it sounds, I've talked to a ton of men who feel almost
jealous of the baby.

And, yes, a lot of men also feel helpless. This whole roller
coaster is as new to them as it is to us, but unlike you, they don't
have a natural role, whether it's feeding the baby or just letting
your battered body heal. That's why it's so helpful if you make
a real effort to draw your partner into the day-to-day caretaking
as much as you can. Even if it's just doing the dishes! It helps
him, it helps you, it helps the whole house, and you're more
of a team. And in the weeks to come, the more the two of you
behave like partners in this new endeavor, the less tired you'll
be, and the faster your sex life will get back to normal (though
don't rush that one, as we'll discuss). It's all connected.

Later on, when the baby's older, you can take more concrete
steps to function not just as a family unit, but as a couple.

When we emerged from that initial haze, Dr. Bickman
started encouraging me to take a weekly date night with Tim.
"My husband and I have gone out every Saturday night since
our first baby was born," she said. "So my kids have no anxiety

Giving specific directions is what works best with my husband. Some men really want to help, but they have no clue what to do. And it's understandable. There's this new baby at home that the mother is taking care of all the time, and they just stand there feeling worthless—which they are, of course. And you need to remember that men for the most part aren't intentionally neglecting all the stuff that needs to get done in the house; they just honestly have NO clue. That's why it's so useful to give them very detailed instructions. Instead of being irritated or simmering in silence, give them concrete guidance. So you say to them, "Please load the dishwasher. Please take out the trash. Please start the laundry. Please go buy wipes. Please order dinner." Whatever needs doing, just spell it out and it'll get done. But if you don't tell them, you can't expect it to just happen magically. My husband is fantastic at following directions. Taking the initiative—not so much. But that's fine. You focus on the baby and let the husband take care of everything else. It will make a big difference in getting you both on the same page.

about what we're doing or when we'll be back—they just expect it. Every single Saturday night, twelve months a year, my husband and I go out together. We might be out for just two hours, but we're out, and that's important for all of us, kids included. There's no anxiety on my end about having to talk to my kids about why we're leaving or where we're going, and there's no anxiety on their end wondering when we're leaving the house and how long we'll be gone and what exact time we'll be back. If it's logistically possible for you, start that tradition as soon as you can. Babies are completely exhausting, and even the most devoted parent in the world doesn't need to have a baby attached to her twenty-four hours a day, seven days a week. Give yourself a break! And, I'll say it again, the babies will be fine if you leave them for two hours! I promise."

It took Tim and me quite a while to get there. Because of our crazy work schedules, we're already gone from Titan more than we'd like, so our idea of a good time is to be with our baby, ogling him and playing with him and just completely obsessing over him. In fact, during one of our very first attempts at a date night after Titan's arrival—he was about two or three months old at the time—we sat down at the restaurant and, before we'd even ordered, we both kept looking underneath the table at our phones. It only took about ten minutes before we realized that we were both stalking Titan on the baby monitor! While we were acting like we were having a good time out on the town, we were both secretly watching Titan at home. We looked at each other, laughed, and said, "All right, time to go home."

At that point, we were just too in love with the baby to miss out on anything, even if it was good for our relationship to be away. Once Titan turned one, we both felt a little bit better about leaving him for an evening so we could take time for just the two of us. And I have to say, finding that time is still a challenge. Between the competing demands of parenthood and our careers, we are still trying to figure out how to carve out dedicated adult-relationship time. I imagine, like so many parents, we're going to be struggling to find that balance for the next several decades.

CHAPTER 20

Will I Ever Get My Groove Back?

(Sex after Baby)

ALL RIGHT, now that you're on the road to reestablishing your connection to your husband, what comes next? Sex should naturally flow from your deep understanding and mutual love of your baby, right? Not so fast.

It took me a long, long time to get back to my old sex life with Tim. First off, I was worried that Tim would want nothing to do with me after watching me give birth. (When it actually went down, he didn't ever look past the blue sheet. He said he didn't *want* to see Titan come out of there—he was afraid he might be too traumatized!) Even so, it was pretty much the least sexy experience ever. My vagina was all beat up and my body just didn't look the same anymore, and especially in those early weeks, I was always hooked up to a breast pump so that I literally looked like a cow in an industrial farm. I was absolutely petrified that Tim would never want to touch me again.

When I brought this fear to Dr. Bickman, she laughed out loud. "Women always think that," she told me. "But have you forgotten who we are talking about? MEN. Women tend to overlook that tiny detail. If he's a man, he won't give a shit. He will want to have sex again instantly. I am talking like five minutes later, in the delivery room, if you let him he would be up for having sex. I recently had this tiny, gorgeous patient who was always perfectly put together and groomed, and then she went into labor. While she was pushing, she kept begging her husband to leave the room. She was completely hysterical about it. 'Don't let him see me, he'll never want to have sex with me again!' she kept screaming. I assured her that was not the case, but she kept telling him to turn around or, if absolutely necessary, to look at her face and not her vaginal opening. But she refused to believe that there was nothing to worry about, that he would still be attracted to her. Three days later, this same patient called me with a different worry: her husband was ready to have sex again and she wasn't!"

That story gave me hope. Tim had always loved the way I looked pregnant, and he loved the baby who'd come out of my huge belly, and he loved *me*, so we would figure it out eventually. In any event, it wasn't like I even wanted to get it on right after pushing a baby out; I just wanted *him* to want it, if you know what I mean. It was almost a relief that I wasn't even allowed to have sex until six weeks after giving birth, until after I'd gone to my postpartum exam. And when that day finally came, I admit to feeling a little nervous. Dr. B. told me that my anxiety was also totally normal: "While women often worry that their partners won't want to have sex with their new bodies again after childbirth, most of the time they come to me at six weeks with the opposite concern—that their husbands want

> I can't tell you how many times I've told women that they're cleared for sex at their six-week visit, only to have them say, "Oh, no, please don't tell my husband that!" That's why I say that you should never, ever, ever bring your husband along on that visit. If he's not in the room, you can tell him whatever you want afterward about when you can have sex again, and he'll never know the difference. Tell him your doctor said six months, or a year! You can make up any time line that suits you. You can say that recovery takes longer after every kid. Again, these are men; you can tell them whatever you want and they will believe you. If you need a little extra time, you take it—and your doctor will back you up.

to have sex but they don't. Many men, surprisingly enough, are ready to go at it way before the six-week clearance, like, say, five minutes after they get home from the hospital. You wouldn't believe how many men have asked me if they could have anal sex because, after all, that hole wasn't the one used to deliver the baby. The Forgotten Hole. That's what I think we should've called this chapter!"

But what if even after six weeks I wasn't ready? Right after Titan was born, I had zero sex drive, and I honestly could not imagine it ever returning. It was hard to feel even remotely in the mood when I was waking up every hour and could barely get through a sit-down meal without wanting to pass out. It was only at three months that I finally felt ready—and I mean *really* ready—to get down to business again.

To my surprise, Tim seemed a little hesitant, which of course made me feel awful. I asked him, "Should I turn out the lights or something? Would it help if you didn't have to look at me?"

Tim was aghast. And because he's also a really good man (hi, honey!), he was also extremely quick to tell me how ridiculous I was being. "Baby, that's not it," he exclaimed. "I'm just terrified of hurting you."

I was flooded with relief, and now it was my turn to reassure him: "Are you kidding me? I just want to have an orgasm!"

I got my wish, but even that wasn't the end of the story. To my surprise, even though my libido had come roaring back, the actual act just didn't feel the same as before. I used to get wet just looking at my husband, but after giving birth it was a little Sahara-like down there, even when I was completely turned on. I had no idea what was wrong with me! Sex didn't hurt exactly, but it just wasn't the same as before.

And, of course, my mind started running through a bunch of what-if questions. Had I not waited long enough to have sex again? Had I further damaged my vajayjay by going at it too soon? Was it always going to feel a little off for the rest of my life? I was concerned enough to speed-dial Dr. Bickman. For the ten millionth time, she told me that a ton of her patients had had the same fears, and that they were for the most part unfounded.

For my own difficulties, Dr. Bickman prescribed me estrogen cream that I used religiously until I was done breastfeeding. I just rubbed it inside my vagina every night for a couple of weeks, and the next time Tim and I had sex, I could really feel the difference. Not totally normal yet, but a lot closer than on our first attempt.

Still, for almost a year after having Titan, long after I'd given up breastfeeding, I didn't get as wet as I had pre-baby and,

There's a reason they call it a "va-dry-na" in the months after you've had a baby. Most women experience extreme vaginal dryness for a while, a result of the low levels of estrogen that are messing with so many other parts of your body as well. It has absolutely nothing to do with the physical state of your vagina! Even if you're quite a few months postpartum, sex might not return to normal until after you're done breastfeeding, since breastfeeding depletes your estrogen and can lead to vaginal dryness. Lower estrogen levels can also atrophy the tissue around your vagina, which can add another layer of discomfort to sex. A lot of people come to me and say, "I had sex too soon, before my vagina had totally healed!' But 99 percent of the time that's not the problem. It's just lower estrogen levels, which will eventually go back to normal. This is the same reason why women who've had C-sections worry about sex not feeling the same after childbirth. If the baby's gigantic head didn't destroy their vaginal opening, what possible reason could there be for painful sex? Hormones, hormones, hormones. So much of what feels so unfamiliar after childbirth has to do with dramatic changes in your body's hormone levels. So even when your vagina is totally healed, the extreme dryness down there can cause serious discomfort during intercourse.

even knowing the medical explanation, I couldn't stop myself from wondering why, if I was so attracted to my husband, my body wasn't reacting like it used to. Was that just the price I was going to pay for having my perfect baby boy? Not that Titan wasn't worth it; I just needed to wrap my head around the new reality if that's what my future held.

But time has a funny way of erasing many of the difficulties of childbirth, and I am happy to report that, as with so many of my postpartum freak-outs, scx finally did return to normal, no estrogen cream necessary. Yes, it took almost a year (I know! You see why I was so worried?), but when we got back on track, we were better than ever before. It was a long wait, but well worth it in the end.

CHAPTER 21

Should I Stay or Should I Go?

(The Return to Work)

THERE COMES A TIME in every mother's life when you have to go back to work, or decide to stay home if you have that option. (Lucky you!) I loved being with Titan so, so much—I still do. I'm completely obsessed with him and part of me never wants to leave his side ever again. But another part of me knows how important it is for my baby to have financial security and all the trappings of a stable life. I want to provide for him to the very best of my abilities. And, yes, doing that requires hard work, and money, and time away from the child. So while I have quite a few friends who decided to become full-time moms after their kids were born, a move I totally respect and admire, I always knew I would be a working mom. In addition to the financial security that's so important to me, I also want to be a career role model for my kids; I hope one day they brag about me (like, hey, the fact that I wrote a book!) when I'm not around.

In any event, when Titan was two months old, I started dipping my toes back into the work world, slowly at first. It felt strange, though, showing up at the studio and feeling like a totally different person—who that was, I wasn't quite sure. As I dashed from meeting to meeting, I kept silently comparing myself to Dorothy in *The Wizard of Oz*—this girl who's just returned from a huge adventure and afterward gets plopped back into the same bedroom, the same bed, with all the same people around me—but I was completely, irrevocably changed by the past two months of my life. And so showing up at the studio again as if no time had passed felt jarring, to say the least. Didn't anyone get how different I was? Didn't anybody see that I was a queen and I'd just had a baby? How could I just go back to work like none of this had happened?

My schedule was also totally screwed up. During my weeks home with Titan, I started to get into the swing of sleeping whenever I could and showering (when I got the chance to shower at all) at the most random hours of the day or night. I was totally focused on feeding and taking care of my new baby, and I lived completely on my own (or rather his) insane schedule. But when I started going back to the studio and taking meetings again, I was still exhausted all the time because trying to adjust to a regular sleep-at-night, wake-during-the-day routine didn't come easy after so many months of snatching bits of sleep here and there. Going back to a relatively normal body clock was hard on me, but it paled in comparison to the difficulty of leaving my son for extended periods.

So, when I was still breastfeeding and pumping around the clock and just couldn't bear to be away from him for more than a few hours, I started taking Titan with me to work. I set up a little travel pack 'n' play where he could take his naps, and

TAKING TIME FOR YOURSELF

Some women can experience serious cabin fever during maternity leave, which makes total sense. You've gone from being out in the world most of your waking hours to lying in bed half-naked with a tiny nonverbal baby all day—of course you feel isolated from time to time! That's why it's really important to get out of the house if you feel like you need it; you don't want to feel like you're stuck in an endless and solitary cycle of feeding and napping and feeding and napping.

Sometimes I would go meet my husband at his office during my leave; it served as a great excuse for me to get dressed, put some makeup on, and drag myself out of the house. Or I'd take the baby to see a movie in the middle of the day—a lot of theaters have mommy-and-me matinees that can be really nice reprieves. The baby sleeps, you can feed him, and most importantly, you're out and about in the world. You could also join a group for new moms in your neighborhood; just getting out of the house to go to the monthly meeting can be great for your sanity.

when I had breaks I would play with him and nurse him and just feel that warm snuggly baby body next to mine. But after a few weeks of this setup, I noticed that Titan wasn't sleeping as well or acting as relaxed when he was out with me—and no wonder! He couldn't smell his smells and hear his sounds and there were people he didn't know milling around. Even at the youngest age, babies know what home is, and I decided that Titan should probably stay there while I was recording.

Though I knew I'd made the right decision for Titan, the separation was so unbearable for me at first—I felt like I was losing a limb when I kissed him goodbye in the morning! I had to go on several short work trips in those first few months of trying to hammer out a new routine, and while I almost always took him with me, sometimes it wasn't possible, and for the first time in my life I felt physically divided. Part of me was at work; the other part of me was at home with my boy. That's still true today. I guess that's just what it is to be a mother.

I faced the biggest of these tests when Titan was just four months old, when I was scheduled to attend Fashion Week in Paris. I was extremely ambivalent about the trip. When I was still pregnant, I was certain that I wanted to go, but of course everything changes when you're actually holding the baby in your arms. You just have no idea how you're going to feel until that happens.

At the time, I was still breastfeeding and in full-on mommy mode, completely focused on Titan, Titan, Titan, Titan from the second I woke up in the morning till I fell exhausted into bed every night. My body was not my own, and even four months on I'd think, "Who the hell is that?" whenever I passed a mirror.

Needless to say, I had my doubts about going on the trip, but I knew I had to do it. Still, I was so worried that my baby would forget about me while I was gone that I took an anxiety pill on the plane. I was just completely bugging.

So, yeah, I was a total mess en route to Paris, but when I got there, something unexpected happened to me. Of course I missed Titan desperately and FaceTimed him constantly, but over the course of that week I started to remember who I was again. I was seeing colors and listening to new music and just feeling really inspired and creatively alive. No less important, I felt *cool* again. For the first time since having Titan, I was more than just a mom, and I liked it. In the end, I got a lot out of taking that little moment for myself. When I got back to L.A., I returned both to parenting and my work with a new vigor. I was so filled up creatively afterward, and I felt so much less guilty about working.

Technology is your friend when it comes to going back to work. Even if you can't be in the same room as your child all the time, you can look at him and make eye contact and see that he's happy, that he's surviving in the world just fine without you right next to him. Whenever I had to be out of the house for more than a few hours, I relied on FaceTime to get my Titan fix, and we also put one of those app-operated cameras in his bedroom so I could spy on him from afar while he slept. There was nothing I loved more than whipping out my phone and catching a glimpse of my sleeping angel! Nest has a particularly awesome system that lets you see the baby clearly and talk to him—all of these tools make it so much easier to leave if you have to.

I even felt, for a beautiful minute or two, like I could juggle the whole shebang. I worked out every day's schedule so that I could get my work in around Titan. Go to the studio, have my meeting, then come back and hang with Titan at lunchtime when he'll definitely be up. Then after he goes back to sleep, I'm going to go back out and tick off all the other items on my never-ending to-do list. That trip definitely helped me get back to that place.

But there are good weeks, and then there are weeks when everything feels completely, crushingly hard, weeks when I feel like I've failed Titan for having to leave the house at all. When I drive away and see him outside playing with his little buddy and he looks up and starts following after the car till I drive out of his line of vision, I feel like I've failed him. I just want to be there every step of the way.

But then, for the hundredth time, I remind myself that he also has to eat and I want him to go to a good school, and I want him to have shoes on his feet, and I want him to have a great place to sleep at night. That reminds me that I haven't failed, that I'm working to contribute to the stability of his childhood. And I also of course know that Titan doesn't need me hovering over him twenty-four hours a day, trying to solve all his problems for him and preventing him from experiencing any real emotional challenges on his own. I know that kind of all-out helicopter parenting would hamper his proper emotional development. But that doesn't mean my heart doesn't break a little every single time I drive away.

This hasn't become any easier as Titan has gotten older. If anything, I'm struggling more than ever to strike the right balance between work and family, and I know I'm not alone. As mothers today, we face so many competing demands— between having a job and having a family, between maintaining relationships with our kids, our spouses, our family members and friends, and bringing in a paycheck—that it can be hard to keep it all straight. How do any of us manage at all? Oh, yeah, because we're superheroes, that's how.

Don't get me wrong, I feel incredibly lucky to have so many

wonderful people and responsibilities in my life but, like almost every mother I know, sometimes I wouldn't mind if my plate were a little less full. And the older Titan gets, and the more life returns to "normal," the harder it is for me to leave him. When he was a baby, I could go to work for a couple of hours and sometimes he'd still be napping when I got home.

But these days, he always realizes in advance when I'm getting ready to go, and he immediately gets really upset. This started right around his first birthday. He'll see me pick up my purse and start crying and reaching for me and grabbing at my pinky finger with his squishy little hand. And even though I think it's rude to be late, and I've always been on time for every meeting or appointment my whole professional life, sometimes I have to sit back down and hold my baby for just a few minutes longer. I'm just not capable of turning my back on my little boy when he's in tears, grasping for me.

Which brings me to another struggle that I'm sure will be familiar to most moms out there. Even though I want to work, I also want to be there for every single moment in my son's life. Of course I understand that's impossible, but I still tear up a little inside whenever I miss any milestone, even the nastier ones. Like this one. The other day when I came home from thirteen straight hours of rehearsing, I opened the front door only to be smacked in the face by this horrible stench. "What *is* that?" I asked my nanny, and she leads me to Titan's room, where he proceeds to go #1 and #2 on his little potty for me. I was so proud of my boy, but I was also really depressed—I couldn't believe I'd missed his first trip to the potty! But at least my nanny saved me the evidence.

FINDING THE RIGHT CAREGIVER

If you do go back to work, you face a million choices. Should you send your child to a day care or a home center? Do you have a relative who can care for him, or do you hire a nanny? We decided on a nanny, and I made a list of qualities that I wanted Titan's caregiver to possess. The first, most important thing was patience, which you can't test out immediately; you have to see someone in action for a while to judge that. I also wanted someone who'd be really gentle with the baby—he was so tiny back then! And lastly, since I travel so much for work, I needed a flexible nanny, someone who could really roll with my sometimes unpredictable schedule. But every family has different needs and different priorities. You just need to take a few minutes to sit down and figure out what yours are.

Dr. Bickman helped me let go of my fear that Titan would forget about me if I left him during the workday. "No matter what," she said, "kids will want you at the end of the day no matter who's been with them since the morning. You're the mom, you're the one who comes first. The most important relationship in their lives is with their parents, period. And while of course it's vitally important to find a loving, responsible caregiver that you respect and trust, your kids will survive when you get a new nanny. I had the same nanny for nine years and she was incredibly important to my family. When she left, I was practically in tears for a week. But my kids? They were completely fine with our new nanny; they didn't even seem to register the transition. Kids are much more resilient than we give them credit for.

CHAPTER 22

When Will Things Go Back to Normal?

(The Rest of Your Life)

IT'S NO SURPRISE that, when you have a baby, your whole world is turned upside down. You're bruised and battered. You feel like you'll never sleep through the night again. You worry that you'll never have sex, or even a *conversation,* with your partner again.

Of course, while that perfect baby makes all these sacrifices worth it, you will occasionally look back on your old body and wonder why you didn't spend your entire life before mother-hood in miniskirts and midriffs, because from now on you'll be dealing with a whole different type of body, a *mother's* body. Your body was built for this magical experience, but that doesn't mean pregnancy and childbirth won't throw it for a major loop. You can get your old shape back if you work for it, but it helps if you accept going into it that, for better or worse, everything will different from now on.

You will also look back on your old life and wonder how you spent your time all those years pre-baby. Because it's true that, as you get the hang of motherhood, more aspects of your pre-baby existence will fall back into place. Your relationships. Your body. Your marriage and sex life. Your work goals. But the busyness—the need to be in three places at once, to be doing eighteen things at the same time—never goes away. If anything, it intensifies as your baby gets older. There are just never enough hours in the day to get it all done.

As my sweet little baby has grown into an active toddler, time has become an even more precious commodity. I constantly feel incomplete without my boy, and all the other necessities of life—like earning a living, and maintaining my friendships, and keeping my household running smoothly—pale in comparison to my constant desire to spend time with my child. No matter what I'm doing, I am always thinking of him. I no longer like being out of town, and I'm always rushing back and forth, trying to get through my day as efficiently as possible so that I can go home and be with him. I'm just completely obsessed with him, and I still have to learn how to have a life away from him.

And, in spite of all the obligations, I didn't want to be *just* a wife and mother. My friendships were also incredibly important to me, and I made an effort to reconnect with my friends after I'd found my footing as a mom, which didn't really happen until around Titan's first birthday. At first I thought my friends, especially the ones who didn't have kids yet, would find me different and duller, but to my surprise we had just as much fun as we'd had in our carefree twenties. Even if I had to go to sleep earlier than I used to, I was pleased to discover

For a lot of the questions I get right after delivery—the broken blood vessels on the face, the darker hair on the mustache line, the bleeding, and of course those wonderful hemorrhoids—I tell patients to wait six weeks and these symptoms will disappear on their own. If they don't, then we'll talk. You might still have pain in certain areas: around your incision site if you've had a C-section, or in your pelvic area if you've had a vaginal birth. Only you can know when pain is mild and normal, and when it requires medical intervention.

Other changes linger longer, though in most cases these, too, are temporary. And, again, if they're not, then your doctor will tell you what you need to be concerned about and what you may just have to roll with. But generally, things *should* get better over time, though that doesn't mean that everything will go back to what it was before. Maybe you have stretch marks, or extra skin at your belly, and that's just how it goes. Love it or hate it, it's just a fact of life.

My rule of thumb is (with the exception of weight loss, which is a more gradual process for some women) that if whatever ails you hasn't gone mostly back to normal within three months, then it probably never will. If you still have a hemorrhoid after three months, you will probably have it for a good long while. If you're still leaking urine after three months, you'll probably be dealing with incontinence for many years to come. I know, but I promise these long-term effects are rare. And, please, just give your body those three months to adjust before you reach any conclusions.

You might not know who you are yet.

that I was still young at heart; if anything, having a baby helped remind me of the joys of childhood.

I am still searching for the perfect balance between motherhood and wifedom and friendship and professional achievement and all the rest of it; I don't think I'll ever feel like I've got everything completely figured out. But which mother does? We all do what we can to get by in one piece.

One of my coping mechanisms, which I've relied on more and more since becoming a mom, is meditation. I'd started to feel as if I was always giving all of my time and energy to the people around me: to my son, to my husband, to my family and friends, and everyone I work with. And while I didn't *mind* that feeling exactly, I decided to make a commitment to take a few minutes every day to step back, breathe in deeply, and collect myself—remember who *I* was. This tiny window of time just for me became a huge pillar of my sanity. Taking those few quiet moments helped me feel calm and centered and capable of taking on the whole juggle.

But of course motherhood is a moving target. Just when you think you have it all figured out, the goalposts move. Your child enters a new phase with new needs, or your job gets more intense, or some unexpected trauma upends your daily routine, as happened when my mother died. You've just got to keep rolling with the constant changes, try to keep your head above water, and ever so occasionally try to enjoy yourself. Your life will be busier, richer, and fuller than ever before, for many years to come. Learn to love the chaos! If you can go easy on yourself, and get over your pre-parenthood perfectionism, and just revel in the miracle of the tiny, amazing creature you made, then you might just be able to enjoy yourself along the way.

INDEX